Coronary Artery Bypass Surgery - New Insights

Edited by Wilbert S. Aronow

Published in London, United Kingdom

Coronary Artery Bypass Surgery - New Insights
http://dx.doi.org/10.5772/intechopen.111004
Edited by Wilbert S. Aronow

Contributors
Amel Hadzimehmedagic, Amgad Mentias, Antonio Nenna, Antonio Salsano, Bagrat G. Alekyan, Bedrudin Banjanovic, Chiara Ferrisi, Edin Kabil, Emir Mujanović, Fasial G. Bakaeen, Francesco Santini, Haytham Elgharably, Jorge Balaguer, Joseph A. Moutiris, José Oliveira, Khaled Ziada, Lejla Divović, Leshya Bokka, Mario Lusini, Massimo Chello, Mehmed Kulić, Mirza Dilić, Muhamed Djedović, Nada Malešić, Narek G. Karapetyan, Nedžad Kadrić, Samed Djedović, Serge C. Harb, Sevleta Avdić, Takashi Murashita, Tarik Selimović, Zina Lazović

First published in London, United Kingdom, 2024 by IntechOpen
IntechOpen is the global imprint of INTECHOPEN LIMITED, registered in England and Wales, registration number: 11086078, 167-169 Great Portland Street, London, W1W 5PF, United Kingdom

British Library Cataloguing-in-Publication Data
A catalogue record for this book is available from the British Library

Additional hard and PDF copies can be obtained from orders@intechopen.com

Coronary Artery Bypass Surgery - New Insights
Edited by Wilbert S. Aronow
p. cm.

This title is part of the Cardiology and Cardiovascular Medicine Book Series, Volume 3
Topic: Cardiovascular Surgery
Series Editor: Kaan Kırali
Topic Editor: Takashi Murashita

Print ISBN 978-1-83769-291-0
Online ISBN 978-1-83769-292-7
eBook (PDF) ISBN 978-1-83769-293-4
ISSN 3033-361X

IntechOpen Book Series

Cardiology and Cardiovascular Medicine

Volume 3

Aims and Scope of the Series

Today, since molecular science on structural causes of oncological pathologies and their molecular treatments are developing at an unbelievable rate, the primary medical cause of death in the twenty-first century will be cardiovascular disease. Neither pandemics that threaten all humanity nor deterioration in the ecosystem will be able to change this fact. Especially, this century seems poised to witness an incredible struggle against atherosclerotic disease, which develops in the arterial walls and results in narrowing and occlusion of the arterial lumen. In addition to this disease, there has been an increasing prevalence of heart rhythm problems, deterioration of heart valves due to aging, and heart failure. Serious vascular pathologies such as stenosis and occlusion, dissection and rupture, and aneurysmal enlargement are also major concerns. Medical and invasive treatment methods may work to save human lives, but they will never provide a real solution. All kinds of medical, technological, and genetic engineering developments obtained in these processes have not yet been sufficient to alleviate or eliminate cardiovascular disease. This book series, Cardiology and Cardiovascular Medicine, includes three topics. The first, Cardiovascular Diseases and Health, reviews important cardiovascular diseases and the developments in their prognosis. The second topic, Cardiovascular Electrophysiology, illuminates the abnormal functioning of the cardiac conduction system, which is caused by all heart pathologies and negatively affects prognosis. The third topic in this series, Cardiovascular Surgery, details treatment for cardiovascular pathologies and how to regulate normal physiological functions with percutaneous or extracorporeal interventions.

Meet the Series Editor

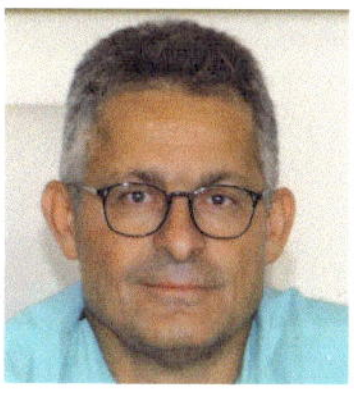

After completing his studies at the Medicine Faculty of Istanbul University in 1990, Prof. Kaan Kırali fulfilled his mandatory medical service and commenced his residency training at Koşuyolu Heart and Research Hospital in 1992. Following five years of assistant education, he pursued further training in England and the USA in 1998. Specializing in laparoscopic and minimally invasive cardiac surgery, he earned the titles of consultant cardiovascular surgeon in 1998, Assistant Professor in 1999, Associate Professor in 2002, and Chief in 2005 at the same hospital. Prof. Kırali also developed an interest in preventive medicine, obtaining an MSc in Public Health from Istanbul University in 2000. Over the past two decades, he has concentrated his scientific pursuits on cardiovascular repairs requiring specialized experience. With his expertise in coronary artery surgery, minimally invasive cardiac surgery, valve repair, and aortic root surgery, he has established new methods for awake coronary bypass revascularization, a new surgical approach for AVR during first and re-operations, aortic valve-sparing procedure, and radiofrequency ablation. Notably, he pioneered awake complete coronary artery bypass grafting (CABG) with bilateral internal mammary arteries (BIMA) and played a crucial role in advancing aortic root surgery with a new aortotomy incision, simplifying aortic valve interventions. Since the year 2000, Prof. Kırali has expanded his interests to heart transplantation, and in recent years, to left ventricular assist devices. He has served as the head of the transplantation department since 2015 and currently continues his work as the director of Koşuyolu High Specialization Education and Research Hospital in Istanbul, Turkey. In his prolific career, he has authored numerous papers in SCI journals, contributed to various book chapters, and served as an editor and reviewer for multiple academic journals. Additionally, he has edited several international books in the field of cardiovascular medicine.

Meet the Volume Editor

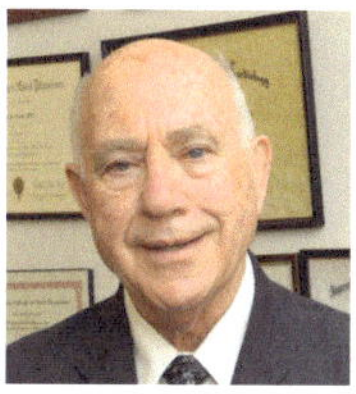

Wilbert S. Aronow, MD, FACC, FAHA, FACP, FCCP, FASPC, AGSF, FGSA is a professor of Medicine and director of Cardiology Research at Westchester Medical Center and New York Medical College. He has edited 22 books and is the author or co-author of 1,753 papers, 212 book chapters in 116 books, 992 commentaries, 50 letters to the editor, and 1,217 abstracts. He has been a member of 185 editorial boards of medical journals. He has been a member of four national guidelines committees. He has been a member of numerous committees of professional societies and a consultant to many government agencies. He is on the lists of best scientists in medicine in the USA and in the world.

Contents

Preface

The book *Coronary Artery Bypass Surgery – New Insights* discusses the latest developments in the management of coronary artery disease. Chapter 1 discusses a multidisciplinary approach to selecting treatment strategies in patients with coronary artery disease and peripheral artery disease. Chapter 2 discusses the perioperative use of Impella 5.5 in patients with high-risk coronary artery bypass grafting. Chapter 3 discusses perioperative ultrasound flow evaluation in grafts and native vessels during coronary artery bypass grafting. Chapter 4 discusses the right ventricular free wall, which is the forgotten territory for coronary revascularization. Chapter 5 discusses an overview of coronary artery surgery with indications and implications for practice. Chapter 6 discusses factors implicated in the clinical follow-up of patients after coronary artery bypass graft surgery. Chapter 7 discusses coronary artery bypass grafting in high-risk patients: on-pump beating-heart CABG. Chapter 8 discusses secondary prevention of coronary artery disease.

I would like to thank all of the authors of these eight excellent chapters for their outstanding work. I would also like to thank you, the reader, for your commitment to providing the best possible care to your patients with coronary artery disease. I hope you will find this book a valuable resource for providing excellent care to your patients with coronary artery disease.

Wilbert S. Aronow, MD, FACC, FAHA
Professor of Medicine and Director of Cardiology Research,
Westchester Medical Center and New York Medical College,
Valhalla, NY, USA

Chapter 1

A Multidisciplinary Approach in Selecting Treatment Strategies in Patients with Aortic and Peripheral Artery Diseases

Bagrat G. Alekyan and Narek G. Karapetyan

Abstract

Coronary artery disease (CAD) is the first leading cause of death worldwide, whereas ischemic stroke due to atherosclerosis of coronary and carotid arteries presents epidemiologically in a different ways among sexes. It ranks the second and the third leading cause of death among women and men globally. Noncoronary atherosclerosis also affects other arterial beds throughout the body, including the aorta and peripheral arteries. Atherosclerosis is a systemic disease affecting all arterial beds, but the progression of atherosclerosis in some arterial beds is triggered by the principal symptoms manifested in one bed and the subclinical course of atherosclerosis in others. There is a high probability of the presence of the so-called polyvascular disease defined as the simultaneous presence of clinically relevant atherosclerotic lesions in at least two arterial beds. It has been shown that patients with cerebral ischemic attacks have a 10-fold higher risk of acute myocardial infarction (AMI) or cardiac death within five years compared to a healthy population. About 35–50% of patients who have undergone carotid endarterectomy (CEA) have severe coronary artery lesions requiring surgical treatment.

Keywords: multidisciplinary approach, peripheral artery diseases, coronary artery disease, Heart Team, multifocal atherosclerosis

1. Introduction

Coronary artery disease (CAD) is the first leading cause of death worldwide, whereas ischemic stroke due to atherosclerosis of coronary and carotid arteries presents epidemiologically in a different ways among sexes. It ranks the second and the third leading cause of death among women and men globally [1, 2]. Noncoronary atherosclerosis also affects other arterial beds throughout the body, including the aorta and peripheral arteries [3, 4]. Atherosclerosis is a systemic disease affecting all arterial beds, but the progression of atherosclerosis in some arterial beds is triggered by the principal symptoms manifested in one bed and the subclinical course of atherosclerosis in others. There is a high probability of the presence of the so-called polyvascular disease defined as the simultaneous presence of clinically relevant atherosclerotic lesions in at least two arterial beds. It has been shown that patients with cerebral ischemic attacks have a 10-fold higher risk of acute myocardial infarction (AMI) or cardiac death within five years compared to a healthy population [5]. About 35–50% of patients who have undergone carotid endarterectomy (CEA) have severe coronary artery lesions requiring surgical treatment [6, 7].

2. The incidence of coronary artery lesions in patients with atherosclerosis of the internal carotid arteries

About 87% of strokes are ischemic, of them 30% are caused by carotid artery atherosclerosis. Moreover, about 10–20% of ischemic strokes are caused by thromboembolism due to atherosclerotic lesions of the internal carotid artery (ICA), and their relative risk increases markedly with stenosis of over 75% [8, 9]. Thus, early detection of atherosclerotic lesions of the internal carotid artery is important for the prevention of ischemic stroke.

The prevalence of concomitant coronary artery disease in ischemic stroke patients varies from 18 to 38%, according to the previously published research [10–13]. The European Society of Cardiology Guidelines on the Diagnosis and Treatment of Peripheral Arterial Diseases reports the incidence of CAD in patients with ICA lesions of 39–61% and of 25 to 72% with the lesions of lower limb arteries (ABI < 0.90) [14].

Timely diagnosis and treatment of concomitant asymptomatic CAD in patients with significant carotid artery lesions can significantly improve the perioperative and long-term results as well as the overall survival rate [15].

Alekyan B.G. et al. assessed 693 patients with atherosclerotic lesions of the internal carotid artery and peripheral arteries admitted to the hospital for selective coronary angiography. A total of 202 (80.5%) patients with isolated atherosclerotic lesions of ICA had at least one coronary artery stenosis of over 50% and 44 (73.3%) patients showed combined atherosclerotic lesions of ICA and lower limb arteries [16].

It is important to note that the SAPPHIRE study is the only multicenter randomized controlled trial (RCT) comparing the results of carotid stenting and CEA in patients with a high surgical risk. The main inclusion criterion was the availability to perform target lesion revascularization, that is, the percutaneous intervention of the target lesion or bypass surgery of the target vessel. The high surgical risk was defined as clinically significant heart disease, severe lung disease, contralateral ICA occlusion or laryngeal nerve palsy, previous radical surgery or radiotherapy on the neck, restenosis after CEA, and age of patients over 80 years.

The SAPPHIRE findings strongly support the role of distal-protected CoC in high-risk patients. Compared with CEA, the rate of cumulative adverse events (death, stroke, ipsilateral stroke, MI) was low and did not differ significantly after 30 days, 1, and 3 years. There were 15 ipsilateral strokes in both groups during the 3-year follow-up. Of them 11 were registered in the carotid stenting group and 9 in the CEA group. Strokes were less frequent at day 30 and after 3 years in the carotid stenting group. The need for target lesion revascularization during the indicated follow-up period did not differ significantly (0.7 vs. 4.6%; $p = 0.04$). Cranial nerve palsy in the carotid stenting group and the CEA group was 0 and 5.3%, respectively ($p = 0.003$) [17].

Alekyan et al. assessed the in-hospital and long-term treatment results of 182 patients with combined coronary and ICA lesions admitted to the hospital in the period from 2017 to 2019. Depending on the treatment strategy, patients were divided into four groups: group 1—staged percutaneous coronary intervention (PCI) and ICA stenting (n = 57 (31.3%)), group 2—staged PCI and CEA (n = 99 (54.4%)), group 3—staged coronary artery bypass grafting (CABG) and ICA stenting (n = 9 (4.9%)), and group 4—simultaneous CABG and CEA (n = 17 (9.4%)). Groups 3 and 4 were excluded from the analysis due to the small number of patients. The in-hospital outcomes in groups 1 and 2 included one death in group 2 after CEA (0 vs. 0.4%, p = 0.44) and one myocardial infarction after PCI (0% vs. 0.4%, p = 0.44). There were one major and minor stroke in each group (p = 0.57). There was no significant difference in the in-hospital outcomes between both groups. The median follow-up was 24.5 months in 87.2% of patients. Twenty (12.8%) patients were lost to follow-up. The primary endpoint of major cardiovascular events occurred in 5 (3.6%) patients. There was one (0.7%) death in group 1. There were no strokes and myocardial infarctions in group 1 during the long-term follow-up. There were two (1.4%) deaths in group 2, one (0.7%) myocardial infarction, and one stroke (0.7%). Deaths from noncardiac and neurological causes were reported in two (1.7%) patients in group 1 and two (1.7%) in group 2. The analysis of the in-hospital and long-term results revealed no significant difference in the incidence of neurological events between the patients who underwent PCI + CEA (group 2) and PCI + ICA stenting (group 1). The individual approach to each patient by a multidisciplinary team, as well as the experience of the operating surgeons, enabled to minimize the possible adverse events [18].

The importance of preoperative diagnosis and revascularization of coronary artery lesions in patients with severe carotid artery lesions was reported by Illuminati et al. [19]. The RCT included 426 patients without prior angina and myocardial ischemic changes according to ECG and Echo-CG. All patients were referred to CEA. The patients were assigned to 2 groups: group A (n = 216) patients underwent coronary angiography and myocardial revascularization before CEA if necessary, and group B (n = 210) underwent only CEA. Significant coronary lesions were diagnosed in 68 (31.5%) patients in group A. Sixty-six patients underwent PCI, and 2 patients underwent simultaneous CEA and CABG. The mean follow-up period was 6.2 years. During the follow-up period, there were three (1.4%) MIs in group A, and 33 (15.7%) in group B ($p < .001$), 6 of which were fatal. At the same time, no myocardial infarctions were reported in group A at 30 days after CEA, whereas there were 9 MIs in group B (p = 0.01), one of which was fatal. The 6.1-year survival rate was 95.6 ± 3.2% in group A and 89.7 ± 3.7% in group B. This study proved that selective coronary angiography followed by myocardial revascularization prior to CEA in patients with asymptomatic coronary artery lesions is safe and can improve long-term survival and freedom from MI [19].

The findings suggest that carotid artery lesion is a predictor of adverse events in both cerebral and coronary circulations, which is a manifestation of systemic atherosclerosis.

Therefore, it is crucial to implement a systemic approach when treating patients with atherosclerosis to obtain adequate stratification of patients with cardiovascular risk factors, as well as to reduce the incidence of adverse events, improve quality of life, and prolong their survival [20].

3. The incidence of coronary artery disease in patients with chronic lower extremity ischemia

The American College of Cardiology and the American Heart Association (ACC/AHA) [21] were among the first to release in 2005 the guidelines on the management of patients with chronic lower limb ischemia. They relied on the previously published studies reporting a high risk of MI, acute impairment of cerebral blood flow, and death in patients with peripheral artery disease. Patients with combined coronary and peripheral artery disease have the risk of CAD-induced death varying from 2 to 6% per year. The risk of MI increases by 20–60% and CABG by 40% in this group of patients.

F.G. Fowkes as well as G.C. Leng et al. [22, 23] demonstrate the importance of outpatient examination for patients with chronic lower limb ischemia and emphasize that patients with asymptomatic (atypical) forms of claudication are more frequently diagnosed with CAD (95% CI 1.3–1.9).

The study by N. Savji et al. included 3.6 million people who underwent obligatory ultrasound examination to detect atherosclerosis of the lower limb arteries. The prevalence of peripheral artery disease was 3.7%. The proportion of patients with at least 2 affected arterial beds increases with age, from 0.04% between 40 and 50 years of age to 3.6% in the 81–90 years age group. Thus, the prevalence of CAD was 2% between 40 to 50 years of age, whereas at 81–90 years, it reached 22.3% ($p < 0.0001$) [24]. The risk of developing MI and CAD increases due to the progression of atherosclerosis [25]. The mortality associated with adverse cardiovascular events such as MI and CHF was higher in patients with chronic lower limb ischemia than in patients with CAD (5.35 vs. 4.52%) at one-year follow-up [25, 26].

During the last decade, many healthcare specialists all over the world have been dealing with the problem of determining a treatment algorithm for patients with chronic lower limb ischemia combined with CAD. Complex treatment of patients reduces the probability of CVD in patients with grade IIB chronic lower limb ischemia, improving the survival and quality of life of patients. The ARIC study [27] reported that male patients with peripheral artery disease were 4–5 times more often diagnosed with CHF compared to patients without arterial lesions of the lower extremities. The available literature indicates that a low ankle-brachial index (<0.9) is indicative of a high prevalence of CAD and CHF. It commonly reflects the presence of generalized atherosclerosis. The above-mentioned data suggest the necessity of preoperative examination of patients with polyvascular disease.

Over the past decade, the number of patients with chronic lower limb ischemia in Europe has increased by 23% [28]. By 2010, the cardiovascular mortality rate increased from 10 to 13 million compared with 1990 [28]. It is closely related to an increase in the prevalence of such risk factors as diabetes mellitus, arterial hypertension, tobacco smoking, and aging [28, 29].

Many studies have shown a high risk of CVD mortality (MI, STEMI) in patients with symptomatic or asymptomatic peripheral artery disease [30]. The ankle-brachial index less than 0.9 doubles the 10-year incidence of coronary events, mortality from cardiovascular events, and overall mortality [31]. About 20% of patients with chronic lower limb ischemia develop MI or CHF 5 years after disease progression with the mortality rate varying from 10 to 15% [32].

The randomized CARP study [33] included 510 patients with chronic lower limb ischemia. The stress test was performed in 74% of patients, and the remaining 26% were consulted by cardiologists. All patients were assigned to two groups: group 1 patients underwent coronary artery revascularization before elective vascular surgery ($n = 258$) and group 2 patients did not undergo coronary artery revascularization before elective vascular surgery ($n = 252$). Coronary angiography was recommended for patients with myocardial ischemia confirmed by the stress test. Patients with the controversial stress test results did not receive coronary angiography. In group 1, 141

(59%) and 99 (41%) patients underwent PCI and CABG, respectively, 8 (3%) patients required urgent vascular intervention, and 9 (3%) patients refused to undergo the intervention. CABG was canceled in one (0.1%) patient due to the development of CHF. The analysis of immediate results showed that 7 (5%) patients in group 1 developed MI after PCI, and 2 (1.4%) had fatal outcomes as a complication of myocardial revascularization. Seven (7.1%) of 99 patients developed MI after PCI and 2 (2.0%) had a fatal outcome. In group 2, where myocardial revascularization was not performed before elective vascular surgery (n = 252), nine (4%) patients underwent coronary artery revascularization in the perioperative period because of unstable angina. During the 30-day follow-up period after lower limb arterial revascularization, there were seven (3%) deaths in the myocardial revascularization group and eight deaths in the group without myocardial revascularization. In group 1, there were two (0.7%) deaths after emergent vascular surgery 7 days after PCI. Thus, a positive outcome from preoperative coronary revascularization was not proven. However, despite the relatively good statistical power of the CARP study, there are some specific limitations. G. Landesberg et al. believe that complete coronary artery revascularization could have prevented postoperative MI and improved survival rate in these patients [34]. Patients were selected for coronary angiography only with a positive stress test result, and patients without anginal complaints who were scheduled for vascular surgery were not screened for pain-free myocardial ischemia.

In 2019, Alekyan B.G. et al. reported that 80.4% of patients with chronic lower limb ischemia had at least one coronary artery lesion of more than 50% among 327 patients undergoing selective coronary angiography [16]. Thus, it can be assumed that in the CARP study a large proportion of patients was underdiagnosed. This argument is confirmed by nine (4%) out of 252 patients who did not undergo myocardial revascularization but required coronary intervention in the postoperative period due to unstable angina pectoris. Importantly, myocardial revascularization was performed in 21 (8%) patients in the long-term follow-up due to the episodes of tension angina [33].

The study of A. Raghunathan et al. reports that MI in 164 patients with chronic lower limb ischemia was the main cause of death. Perioperative MI was observed in 10 (12.4%) of 84 patients who underwent myocardial revascularization, whereas among those who did not undergo myocardial revascularization (n = 80) perioperative MI was defined in 18 (21.7%) patients. In the long-term period, one (1.2%) and two (2.4%) patients died, respectively. Importantly, 41 (25%) patients developed acute MI in the long-term follow-up [35].

A prospective randomized study by M. Monaco et al. with a study population of 208 patients with obstructive aortoiliac segment lesions and aortic aneurysms demonstrates a positive effect of coronary angiography and myocardial revascularization on long-term outcomes [36]. All the patients were divided into two groups. Group 1 (n = 103, 49.5%) patients underwent the stress test with the subsequent coronary angiography if required. Group 2 included 105 (50.4%) patients who underwent coronary angiography before vascular surgery. Forty-seven (45.6%) of 103 patients in group 1 who were referred to selective coronary angiography had positive stress test results. According to coronary angiography findings, significant coronary artery stenoses were detected in 46 (97.8%) patients. Myocardial revascularization was performed in 42 (91.3%) patients, among whom 1 (2.4%) died due to the cardiogenic shock. Three (7.1%) of 42 patients did not undergo vascular surgery and two (4.7%) patients refused to undergo it. Thirty-eight (90.5%) of 42 patients underwent elective lower extremity revascularization within 2 months. No fatal outcomes were recorded.

The remaining 61 (59.2%) patients with a negative stress test result underwent elective vascular surgery without preoperative coronary angiography. There were five (8.2%) fatal outcomes from cardiovascular complications in this subgroup.

Sixty-five (61.9%) of 105 patients in group 2, who underwent coronarography, had significant coronary artery lesions. There were no complications associated with coronary angiography. Coronary artery revascularization was performed in 61 (93.8%) of them. The overall incidence of major cardiovascular complications in the in-hospital period, including cardiac mortality, was higher in group 1 (11.6%) patients than in group 2 (4.7%; $p = 0.1$). Freedom from cardiovascular events at the end of the 4-year follow-up was 69.6 ± 4.7% in group 1 and 86.6 ± 3.6% in group 2 with an absolute risk reduction of 16.7% corresponding to a relative risk reduction of 59.4% (95% CI 1.4–6.8; $p = 0.04$). Event freedom at 8 years was 53.5 ± 6.3% in group 1 and 77.5 ± 4.8% in group 2 with an absolute risk reduction of 19.8% corresponding to a relative risk reduction of 53.6% (95% CI 1.4–5.7; $p = 0.002$). The authors concluded that coronary angiography followed by coronary artery revascularization reduces the risk of cardiovascular events in these patients.

The consensus published by the American College of Cardiology, American Heart Association, Society of Cardiovascular Angiography and Intervention, and Society of Interventional Radiologists in 2018 confirmed that patients with intermittent claudication associated with the lesions in the aortoiliac, femoral, and patellar segments and tibial arteries and failure of conservative therapy should be considered for endovascular treatment [37]. This consensus also emphasizes the importance of diagnosing lesions in other arterial beds, including coronary arteries, to reduce high morbidity and mortality in patients with chronic lower limb ischemia. Endovascular and surgical lower extremity revascularization plays a crucial role in reducing mortality. Thus, the mortality rate reaches 20% within 6 months and 50% within 5 years in patients who remain without proper treatment [37].

4. Incidence of coronary artery lesions in patients with critical lower limb ischemia

The main cause of death in patients with peripheral arterial disease is coronary artery disease [14, 38, 39]. Critical lower limb ischemia is an aggressive form of systemic atherosclerosis and is the most common cause of amputation [36, 40, 41]. Due to the prevalence of atherosclerosis, diabetes mellitus, and smoking, patients with critical lower limb ischemia have a high risk of cardiovascular events, including death.

The worldwide prevalence of peripheral arterial disease, according to various authors, ranges from 3 to 10% in the general population and is increasing with aging, nutritional errors, and high incidence of diabetes mellitus [42–44]. Peripheral arterial disease is often associated with atherosclerotic diseases such as CAD or ICA lesions. A high prevalence of CAD in patients with peripheral arterial disease has been reported [45, 46].

The high-risk group of patients with peripheral arterial disease is the group of patients with critical lower limb ischemia, commonly present with ischemic rest pain in the foot or ankle and/or the presence of trophic ulcers or non-healing wounds. The prevalence of critical lower limb ischemia is estimated at 500 to 1000 cases per million people annually. Given the aging population, the global increase in metabolic syndrome, the burden of diabetes mellitus and tobacco smoking, the prevalence of both peripheral arterial disease and critical lower limb ischemia is projected to increase [46, 47].

Critical lower limb ischemia is associated with significant disability and mortality. Since its diagnosis in patients without limb revascularization, amputation is required in 20–40% of patients within 6 months and less than 80% of patients survive [19, 39, 48]. A large German registry reported that critical lower limb ischemia was associated with the 4-year amputation rate of 35–67% and the related mortality rate of 52–64% [49].

The large REACH registry included 68,236 patients with various arterial bed lesions. All the study population was divided into four groups: those who had risk factors but no verified arterial lesions (n = 11,587), those who had lesions of one arterial bed (n = 42,716), two arterial beds (n = 9542), and three arterial beds (n = 1132). The study was aimed at assessing the incidence of cardiovascular events in patients with atherosclerosis within the 12-month follow-up. Patients with isolated lower limb arterial lesions had fewer cardiovascular complications and deaths than patients with polyvascular disease, including those with concomitant CAD [50–53].

In 2019, Alekyan B.G. et al. analyzed the data of 398 patients with peripheral artery disease admitted to the hospital for elective revascularization surgery within the 20-month period. According to the study protocol, all patients underwent selective coronary angiography to visualize the coronary bed. The treatment strategy of each patient was individually discussed with the Heart Team to select the optimal revascularization strategy. The authors concluded that 320 (80.4%) of 398 patients had at least one coronary artery stenosis over 50%. Of them, 177 (55.3%) patients underwent direct myocardial revascularization (93%—PCI and 7%—CABG). Patients with combined lesions of coronary and lower limb arteries and absolute contraindications to cardiac stress testing should undergo coronary artery imaging (MSCT, coronary angiography) to choose the optimal treatment strategy [16]. These findings are consistent with the previous study performed by Pokrovsky A.V. and Dogujeva R.M. in 2012. All patients underwent open surgery without prior coronary angiography and myocardial revascularization. The mean follow-up was 62.04 ± 1.23 months. The long-term results of treatment were evaluated in patients after reconstructive surgery for Leriche syndrome combined with diabetes mellitus. In 63.5% of patients, the main cause of death was MI in the long-term period. The authors concluded that coronary imaging is required before elective lower extremity revascularization. Prevention of cardiovascular events ensures the reduction of cardiovascular complications in patients with Leriche syndrome [16].

Chen C. et al. included 879 patients with chronic and critical lower limb ischemia who underwent lower extremity revascularization. All the patients were enrolled into two groups: patients with 2B chronic lower limb ischemia (n = 382 (43.4%)) and patients with critical lower limb ischemia (n = 497 (56.5%)). Two subgroups were allocated within each group: isolated chronic lower limb ischemia (n = 177 (46.3%)) and chronic lower limb ischemia and CAD (n = 205 (53.6%)) versus isolated critical lower limb ischemia (n = 246 (49.4%)) and critical lower limb ischemia and CAD (n = 251 (50.0%)). Major adverse cardiovascular and cerebrovascular events (MACCE) and all-cause mortality during 5 years of follow-up were evaluated. Patients with critical lower limb ischemia and CAD were more likely to receive medication therapy (aspirin, DAATs, beta blockers, and statins). In addition, they were older, more likely to have hypertension, heart failure, diabetes mellitus, and renal failure compared with the group with isolated critical lower limb ischemia. The subanalysis of the critical lower limb ischemia + CAD group reported that these patients had the worst rates of both, MACCE, and all-cause mortality after 5 years, compared to patients with isolated critical lower limb ischemia. Patients with critical lower limb ischemia and CAD demonstrated a fourfold increased incidence of MACCE as well as all-cause mortality after 5 years compared to patients with chronic lower limb ischemia and CAD.

The association between CAD and adverse long-term clinical outcomes was stronger in patients with isolated critical lower limb ischemia. MACCE and mortality rates increased by 52 and 64% in patients with critical lower limb ischemia and CAD, compared to patients with isolated critical lower limb ischemia [52, 53].

Nishijima A. et al. retrospectively studied the prevalence of CAD in 129 patients with critical lower limb ischemia who underwent lower limb amputation. Patients were divided into two groups: group 1 had major amputation above the ankle (n = 36) and group 2 had minor amputation below the ankle or necrotomy (n = 93). Selective coronary angiography was performed in 93.7% of patients with critical lower limb ischemia. Coronary artery lesions were detected in 69% of patients. A more detailed analysis revealed that 82% of patients who underwent major amputations had coronary artery lesions, whereas in the group with minor amputations the prevalence rate reached 63%. Thus, the authors proved that patients who underwent major amputations had a significantly higher prevalence of CAD compared to those patients who underwent minor amputations. In addition, the data of patients without critical lower limb ischemia (566 patients with grade 2B chronic lower limb ischemia) were reviewed. They underwent endovascular lower extremity revascularization. According to coronary angiography, only 40% (227 out of 566) of them had CAD [54].

The study of Soga Y. et al. evaluated the survival rate of 995 patients with critical lower limb ischemia within 2 years after endovascular lower extremity revascularization. The 2-year mortality rate was 41.4% (n = 412). The causes of death included cardiac events (n = 121, 29%), vascular events (n = 41, 10%), sudden death (n = 32, 8%), noncardiovascular events (n = 191, 46%), and unexplained causes (n = 27, 7%). Notably, 47% (194 of 412) of all deaths were due to cardiovascular causes. Heart failure was the most common cause of death in the cardiac mortality group (37.1%). Acute myocardial infarction (22.3%) and ventricular fibrillation (9.9%) ranked second and third, respectively. Thus, treatment of heart failure and prevention of ischemic complications are important for patients with critical lower limb ischemia. Sepsis, pneumonia, and cancer were the most frequent causes of noncardiovascular deaths. About 34% (n = 142) died due to infectious diseases [55].

The presence of CAD may be underestimated in patients with critical lower limb ischemia since they often suffer from diabetic neuropathy and/or physical inactivity due to rest pain or trophic ulcers. Therefore, these patients do not complain of typical heart pain. Helzer N.R. et al. evaluated coronary angiograms before vascular surgery in 300 patients with critical lower limb ischemia and showed that only 8% of patients had mild coronary artery stenoses [56].

Current evidence state that myocardial ischemia should be assessed in patients with critical lower limb ischemia [16, 33, 54]. However, there is no consensus on the screening method for determining myocardial ischemia in this group of patients. Patients with critical lower limb ischemia may not report cardiac complaints (angina and dyspnea) due to their physical inactivity. In addition, the prevalence of diabetes mellitus in patients with critical lower limb ischemia ranges from 75 to 83%, and therefore, clinical signs of angina may sometimes be underestimated, given the development of pain-free myocardial ischemia in patients [57, 58]. According to the 2019 ESC guidelines for the diagnosis and treatment of chronic coronary syndromes, when CAD cannot be excluded by clinical assessment of disease symptoms, noninvasive diagnostic tests should be considered to confirm the diagnosis and assess the risk of fatal events in the future. Noninvasive methods of myocardial ischemia imaging (scintigraphy, PET/CT) or coronary bed imaging using MSCT coronary angiography should be applied [59].

The role of coronary revascularization in patients with peripheral artery disease requiring vascular revascularization was assessed in the CARP study on 510 patients. Group 1 patients underwent coronary artery revascularization before lower extremity revascularization (n = 258). Group 2 patients were not referred to coronary artery revascularization (n = 252).

Coronary angiography was performed only in patients with a positive stress test. Patients with controversial results were not referred to coronary angiography. Preoperative coronary revascularization was not proven to be beneficial according to the results of the study. There were no significant differences in the incidence of myocardial infarction, mortality, or the length of the in-hospital stay when assessing the immediate results. There were 7 (3.1%) deaths in the myocardial revascularization group versus 8 (3.4%) deaths in the group without revascularization ($p = 0.87$). A total of 19 (8.4%) patients in the myocardial revascularization group had acute myocardial infarction (AMI) versus 20 (8.4%) without myocardial revascularization ($p = 0.99$). CHF leading to fatal outcomes was registered in one (0.4%) patient in the myocardial revascularization group versus two (0.8%) patients without myocardial revascularization ($p = 0.59$). In the long-term follow-up period, patients with and without myocardial revascularization had similar mortality rates after 2.6 years (22 vs. 23%). Among the patients who did not undergo preoperative coronary artery revascularization, 21 (8%) underwent coronary artery revascularization after lower extremity revascularization [33].

The CARP study was criticized by several researchers, who pointed out its significant limitations. Thus, Landesberg G. and Kertai M believe that complete myocardial revascularization in this group of patients could prevent postoperative AMI cases and could improve long-term survival rates [60].

Coronary angiography and myocardial revascularization in the CARP study were performed only in patients with confirmed myocardial ischemia using cardiac stress testing. Thus, the patients who had no complaints of cardiac pain did not undergo revascularization. Alekyan B.G. et al. showed that 66.4% of patients with chronic lower limb ischemia and critical lower limb ischemia with concomitant CAD are asymptomatic despite the presence of at least one coronary artery lesion of over 50% [16]. It means that a large proportion of patients in the CARP study could have severe coronary artery lesions. A total of 4% of patients who did not undergo myocardial revascularization were subjected to myocardial revascularization due to ACS in the in-hospital period. Moreover, 8% of patients who did not undergo myocardial revascularization before elective vascular surgery were referred to it due to the clinical symptoms in the long-term period [33].

In addition to the above-mentioned limitations of the CARP study, it is worth considering that 16 years have passed since the results of the study were presented. During this time, new endovascular technologies appeared, including new generation of stents, myocardial fractional flow reserve, various intracoronary imaging methods (intravascular ultrasound and optical coherence tomography), etc. These novel technologies may question the relevance and reliability of the presented findings.

Raghunathan A. et al. performed the subanalysis of the CARP study, which included 143 patients with critical lower limb ischemia. All these patients had concomitant CAD. Then, they were randomized into two groups: group 1 patients underwent myocardial revascularization before elective lower extremity revascularization (n = 61, of them 28 patients underwent CABG and 33 patients—PCI) and group 2 patients who did not undergo myocardial revascularization (n = 82). The immediate and long-term results were assessed using the incidence of MACCE. The 30-day overall mortality in patients with critical lower limb ischemia and CAD was 3.5% (n = 5). Three (4.9%) patients died in 1st group, and in 2nd group died 2 (2.4%) (p = 0.42). The incidence of MI in the in-hospital period was 8.4% (4.6% in group 1 vs. 11.5% in group 2; p = 0.19). The 2.7-year overall survival was 79% and the incidence of AMI was 16.1%. The authors concluded that AMI was the main cause of death in these patients. Coronary angiography and subsequent myocardial revascularization in this group of patients could have prevented possible acute myocardial infarction [35].

Several authors note that the incidence of diabetes mellitus (70.4%), chronic renal failure (27.8%), and smoking (70 to 90%) is higher in patients with critical lower limb ischemia compared to patients with chronic lower limb ischemia. These risk factors significantly increase the risk of developing adverse cardiovascular events, including mortality, acute cerebrovascular events, and acute myocardial infarction [57, 61–63].

At 1 year, 25% of patients with critical lower limb ischemia without coronary artery imaging will be dead and 30% will have undergone amputation. Only 45% will remain alive with both limbs. At 5 years, over 60% of patients with critical limb ischemia will be dead mainly from myocardial infarction or stroke [46, 61, 64, 65].

Taking into account that patients with critical lower limb ischemia have a high risk of cardiovascular complications, routine coronary angiography, and subsequent myocardial revascularization, if indicated, seems to be reasonable and rationale.

5. Multidisciplinary approach in the treatment of patients with peripheral arterial disease

The treatment of CAD in patients with coexisting peripheral arterial disease referred to endovascular or surgical lower extremity revascularization remains challenging. The accurate diagnosis of atherosclerotic lesions in all arterial beds and the optimal strategy of treatment are critical for these patients. Therefore, a multidisciplinary team should involve different healthcare specialists.

The multidisciplinary approach emerged in oncology in the 1960s and demonstrated its effectiveness in improving the treatment outcomes of cancer patients [66, 67]. Concerning myocardial revascularization this approach has been offered after several large randomized trials with the SYNTAX study to be the first one. The multidisciplinary approach has received a class 1C recommendation in the ESC guidelines on myocardial revascularization since 2010 [48]. But in case of combined coronary and peripheral artery lesions, this approach has not been widely used so far. The multidisciplinary approach in the treatment of patients with aortic and peripheral artery disease who should undergo preoperative CAD assessment was first mentioned in the ESC guidelines on non-cardiac surgery [68]. Preoperative myocardial revascularization should be performed in patients with proven myocardial ischemia and CAD risk factors, including angina, a positive history of postinfarction cardiosclerosis, heart failure, prior STEMI or TIA, renal dysfunction, and the presence of diabetes mellitus. If patients have at least two risk factors, it is recommended to perform preoperative stress testing or coronary imaging (Class II a). Recent ESC guidelines on peripheral artery diseases [69] have already indicated the need for using the multidisciplinary team for joint decision-making on the treatment of these patients.

Coexisting CAD should be confirmed in patients with peripheral artery disease. But it remains challenging in those patients who have absolute contraindications for cardiac stress testing (Leriche syndrome, prior stroke, and intermittent claudication). The second important issue is the necessity to choose the optimal strategy and staging of coronary and peripheral arterial bed revascularization.

6. Methods

A total of 693 patients with aortic and peripheral artery diseases admitted to the A.V. Vishnevsky National Medical Research Center of Surgery for elective revascularization were enrolled in the period from May 1, 2017 to December 31, 2018 (over 20 months).

The study protocol was approved by the Local Ethics Committee. The multidisciplinary team referred all patients to selective coronary angiography to identify the severity of coronary artery lesions and determine the optimal strategy for coronary and peripheral artery revascularization.

The exclusion criteria were as follows: acute coronary syndrome, acute peripheral artery thrombosis, renal failure, previously performed selective coronary angiography, or cardiac stress testing.

A significant coronary lesion on angiography was defined as a luminal narrowing with a diameter stenosis of more than 50%, and hemodynamically significant was defined as a luminal narrowing with a diameter stenosis of more than 75% or a lesion of less than 75%, but with proven myocardial ischemia.

The primary endpoints were AMI, STEMI, and death. The secondary endpoints included access site complications, bleeding, infections, and stroke.

A total of 693 patients with aortic and peripheral artery disease were recruited to the study. Of them, 171 (32.5%) were women and 522 (75.3%) were men. The age of the patients ranged from 29 to 93 years with the mean age of 67.2 ± 8.8 years. 32.5% (n = 223) of patients were over 71 years of age.

Only 203 (29.3%) patients had cardiac complaints, whereas 490 (70.7%) were asymptomatic. The majority of patients had isolated ICA lesion (n = 196, 28.3%). A total of 93 (13.4%) patients had combined ICA and lower extremity artery lesions, 70 (10.1%) patients were present with combined iliac and superficial femoral artery lesions, and 60 (8.6%) patients were with femoral artery lesions.

7. Results

Selective coronary angiography revealed that 554 (79.9%) patients out of 693 had at least one coronary artery lesion of more than 50%. Importantly, 368 (66.4%) of these patients were clinically asymptomatic and had no cardiac complaints (**Table 1**). About 80.5% of patients with isolated ICA lesion (n = 251) and 81.6% of patients with isolated lower extremity artery lesion (n = 327) had over 50% stenosis of at least one coronary artery (**Table 2**).

Single-vessel, double-vessel, and triple-vessel coronary artery disease of more than 50% were found in 174 (31.4%), 140 (25.3%), and 135 (24.4%) patients, respectively. The left main coronary artery disease was found in 88 (15.9%) patients.

A comparative analysis of the CAD incidence showed that 314 (77.0%) patients with a single arterial bed lesion had stenoses of more than 50%. The incidence of

Heart complaints	Presence of coronary artery lesions				Total	%
	< 50%		> 50%			
	n	%	n	%		
Symptomatic	17	12.2	186	33.6	203	29.3
Asymptomatic	122	87.8	368	66.4	490	70.7
Total	139	100	554	100	693	100

Table 1.
Distribution of patients with peripheral arterial disease according to the CAD symptoms and signs.

Nature of peripheral arterial lesions	Presence of coronary artery lesions > 50%		Total
	n	%	
Isolated lesion of the lower extremity arteries	267	81.6	327
Isolated ICA lesion	202	80.5	251
Internal carotid arteries and lower extremities	44	73.3	60
Aortic aneurysms	22	68.8	32
Brachiocephalic arteries and lower extremities	9	81.1	11
Visceral and renal arteries	6	85.7	7
Brachiocephalic arteries	4	80.0	5
Total	554	79.9	693

Table 2.
Incidence of coronary artery stenoses of more than 50% in patients with peripheral artery disease.

CAD increased with the number of affected peripheral arterial beds. Atherosclerotic lesions of at least two arterial beds were associated with the stenoses of more than 50% ranging from 83.2 to 89.3%. The incidence of CAD increases with the number of affected arterial beds.

After coronary angiography, all patients were discussed by the multidisciplinary Heart Team to choose the optimal treatment strategy and staging for both myocardial and lower extremity revascularizations.

A total of 238 (43.0%) patients with at least one coronary artery stenosis of more than 50% did not undergo myocardial revascularization. Seventeen (3.0%) patients were referred to additional examination to verify myocardial ischemia. 221 (40.0%) patients had no indications for revascularization. A total of 316 (57.0%) patients underwent myocardial revascularization according to the decision of the multidisciplinary team. Twenty-one (6.7%) patients underwent CABG and 295 (50.3%)—PCI. Thus, a total of 45.6% (n = 316) of patients underwent myocardial revascularization by the multidisciplinary team decision. About 57.0% of patients with at least one coronary artery stenosis of more than 50% underwent myocardial revascularization.

A total of 295 patients underwent staged PCIs. Eighty-one (27.5%) and 79 (26.8%) patients underwent the LAD and RCA stenting, respectively. Thirty-nine (13.2%) patients underwent the LAD + RCA stenting, and 17 (5.7%) patients underwent

LMCA stenting. All patients were implanted with the latest generation of the antiproliferative drug-eluting stents (the mean of 1.7 stents per patient).

A total of 207 (29.9%) of 693 patients were not referred to vascular surgery according to the multidisciplinary team decision. Eighteen (8.7%) patients were referred to additional examinations, and 40 (19.3%) patients were prescribed optimal medication therapy. Eighty-three (40.1%) did not return to the hospital for surgery, and 66 patients were discharged for the final stage of intervention.

Surgical and endovascular surgeries for aortic and peripheral artery disease were performed in 486 (70.1%) patients. Myocardial revascularization was performed in 226 (46.5%) patients in addition to vascular surgery, while no myocardial revascularization was performed in 260 (53.5%). Of 226 patients, 214 (94.7%) underwent PCI and 12 (5.3%) underwent CABG. A total of 486 patients underwent 509 vascular surgeries: 341 (67.0%) underwent surgical lower extremity revascularization, 165 (32.4%)—endovascular lower extremity revascularization, and 3 (0.6%)—hybrid revascularization.

As for the strategy for CAD treatment in patients with aortic and peripheral artery disease, myocardial revascularization was performed in 50% of patients who underwent CEA (47.3%—PCI, 2.7%—CABG) and in 51.3% of patients (50%—PCI, 1.3%—CABG) who underwent open surgery in the aorto-femoral segment, and in 66.7% of patients (66.7%—PCI) who underwent ICA stenting.

A total of 923 (564 endovascular and 359 surgical) interventions were performed in 580 patients. Three (0.51%) patients died in the in-hospital period. Hemorrhagic stroke provoked by the hypertensive crisis after successful PCI was the cause of one (0.17%) death. Two other patients (0.34%) died because of hemorrhagic and ischemic strokes after CEA. Two (0.56%) patients had stroke: one patient after ICA grafting and one patient after CEA. There were no cases of acute myocardial infarction in the in-hospital period in both groups. Among the secondary endpoints, hematomas in the postoperative wound area after open interventions occurred in 2 (0.56%) cases, vascular conduit infections in 2 (0.56%), and hemopericardium after PCI in 1 case that did not require pericardiocentesis.

8. Conclusion

Our results demonstrated that 79.9% (n = 558) of patients with atherosclerotic lesions of the aorta and peripheral arteries had at least one coronary artery stenosis of more than 50% according to selective coronary angiography. The relationship between the number of the affected coronary arteries with stenoses of over 50.0% and the number of affected arterial beds has been found. The more arterial beds are affected, the more coronary arteries are affected. The prevalence of CAD reaches almost 90%, when four or more peripheral arterial beds are affected. About 66.4% of patients with aortic and peripheral arterial disease and coexisting coronary artery stenosis of more than 50% were asymptomatic.

Importantly, 316 (45.6%) out of 693 patients with aortic and peripheral artery diseases had hemodynamically significant coronary artery stenoses, requiring direct myocardial revascularization (295—PCI and 21—CABG). Combined significant aortic lesions, peripheral artery disease, critical lesions of the carotid arteries, as well as other comorbidities were the main reasons for the refusal of CABG in some patients with severe CAD and the Syntax Score over 23.

Out of 398 staged PCIs, 295 patients had only one (0.34%) fatal outcome associated with hemorrhagic stroke caused by uncontrolled arterial hypertension. Taking into account the low incidence of in-hospital complications following PCI, we may consider that PCI is the method of choice for treating this group of patients.

We agree with the current guidelines suggesting first to collect patients' medical history and complaints to define possible coronary artery stenosis. If a patient is likely to have CAD, noninvasive stress testing is recommended with the subsequent referral to intracoronary imaging (CT or invasive coronary angiography). However, we face some challenges in the real clinical practice that we should keep in mind. A large proportion of patients have absolute contraindications for cardiac stress testing (symptomatic ICA lesion, stroke, and chronic and critical lower limb ischemia) and socio-economic limitations (lack of availability of stress testing and myocardial scintigraphy in most hospitals, and the out-of-pocket expenses for patients to undergo additional testing). In addition, the results of noninvasive stress testing do not necessarily correspond to angiographic findings. Patel et al. have previously shown important relationships between the clinical profile of patients, findings after noninvasive stress testing, and the absence of coronary artery stenoses according to selective coronary angiography on 661,063 patients from 1128 hospitals in the USA. The patients were divided into two groups according to the presence or absence of significant coronary artery atherosclerotic lesions. As a result, 37.6% of patients who did not undergo stress testing before coronary angiography had CAD. About 33.7% patients with controversial stress testing results had CAD. About 30% of patients with negative stress testing results had coronary obstructions [70].

When noninvasive testing to confirm CAD is unavailable, we should use other options to detect it. The results of our study have shown a high prevalence (79.9%) of coronary atherosclerosis in patients with aortic and peripheral artery diseases, as well as the resultant high rate of myocardial revascularization (45.7%).

Out of 923 endovascular and surgical interventions performed on 580 patients in the in-hospital period, three (0.51%) patients died, and two (0.34%) patients experienced AMI. This indicates the high efficiency and safety of the multidisciplinary approach in the treatment of CAD patients with aortic and peripheral artery diseases. None of the patients had ACS in the in-hospital period, confirming the accurate preoperative assessment of coronary artery disease and the optimal decision on PCI and CABG.

We have previously published in-hospital outcomes of endovascular treatment of patients with combined coronary and ICA lesions, showing high efficacy and safety of the complex treatment and complete revascularization of both carotid and coronary arterial beds with complete absence of both fatal outcomes and acute myocardial infarction and stroke among these patients [16]. According to the secondary endpoints, the following complications were registered in four (12.9%) patients: One (3.2%) patient had radial artery thrombosis after PCI, two (6.5%) were diagnosed with pulsatile hematoma of the access site (common right femoral artery) after ICA stenting. All these complications were treated conservatively.

The treatment strategy for patients with polyvascular disease should include both, accurate assessment of all arterial beds prior to the intervention and treatment of all, even clinically unapparent, significant lesions of the remaining segments.

Conflict of interest

The authors declare no conflict of interest.

Author details

Bagrat G. Alekyan[1] and Narek G. Karapetyan[2]*

1 RAS Academician, Center for Endovascular Surgery at the A.V. Vishnevsky Scientific Research Center, Moscow, Russian Federation

2 Center for Endovascular Surgery at the A.V. Vishnevsky Scientific, Moscow, Russian Federation

*Address all correspondence to: ngkarapetyan@gmail.com

References

[1] OECD. Health at a Glance 2017: OECD Indicators. Paris: OECD Publishing; 2017. DOI: 10.1787/health_glance-2017-en

[2] Geleijnse JM. Global, regional, and national age sex specific all-cause and cause specific mortality for 240 causes of death, 1990 - 2013: A systematic analysis for the global burden of disease study 2013. Lancet. 2015;**385**:117

[3] Mendis S, Puska P, Norrving BE. Global atlas on cardiovascular disease prevention and control. Geneva: World Health Organization (WHO); 2011. Available from: https://www.who.int/cardiovascular_diseases/publications/atlas_cvd/en/

[4] Nichols M, Townsend N, Luengo-Fernandez R, et al. European Cardiovascular Disease Statistics. Brussels: European Heart Network; 2012 (European Society of Cardiology, Sophia Antipolis). Available from: https://www.escardio.org/static_file/Escardio/Press-media/press-releases/2013/EU-cardiovascular-disease-statistics-2012.pdf

[5] Nadareishvili ZG, Rothwell PM, Beletsky V, Pagniello A, Norris JW. Long-term risk of stroke and other vascular events in patients with asymptomatic carotid artery stenosis. Archives of Neurology. 2002;**59**(7):1162-1166

[6] Hertzer NR, O'hara PJ, Mascha EJ, Krajewski LP, Sullivan TM, Beven EG. Early outcome assessment for 2228 consecutive carotid endarterectomy procedures: The Cleveland clinic experience from 1989 to 1995. Journal of Vascular Surgery. 1997;**26**(1):1-10

[7] Salasidis GC, Latter DA, Steinmetz OK, Blair JF, Graham AM. Carotid artery duplex scanning in preoperative assessment for coronary artery revascularization: the association between peripheral vascular disease, carotid artery stenosis, and stroke. Journal of Vascular Surgery. 1995;**21**(1):154-162

[8] Amato M, Montorsi P, Ravani A, Oldani E, Galli S, Ravagnani PM, et al. Carotid intima-media thickness by B-mode ultrasound as surrogate of coronary atherosclerosis: Correlation with quantitative coronary angiography and coronary intravascular ultrasound findings. European Heart Journal. 2007;**28**(17):2094-2101

[9] Gopaldas RR et al. Staged versus synchronous carotid endarterectomy and coronary artery bypass grafting: Analysis of 10-year nationwide outcomes. The Annals of Thoracic Surgery. 2011;**91**(5):1323-1329

[10] Aichner FT, Topakian R, Alberts MJ, Bhatt DL, Haring HP, Hill MD, et al. High cardiovascular event rates in patients with asymptomatic carotid stenosis: The REACH registry. European Journal of Neurology. 2009;**16**(8):902-908

[11] Benjamin EJ, Muntner P, Bittencourt MS. Heart disease and stroke statistics-2019 update: A report from the American Heart Association. Circulation. 2019;**139**(10):56-528

[12] Gansevoort RT, Correa-Rotter R, Hemmelgarn BR, Jafar TH, Heerspink HJL, Mann JF, et al. Chronic kidney disease and cardiovascular risk: Epidemiology, mechanisms, and prevention. Lancet. 2013;**382**(9889):339-352

[13] Tsao CW, Aday AW, Almarzooq ZI, Alonso A, Beaton AZ, et al. Heart disease and stroke statistics-2022 update: A report from the American heart association. Circulation. 2022;**145**(8):e153-e639. DOI: 10.1161/CIR.0000000000001052. Epub 2022 Jan 26. Erratum in: Circulation. 2022 Sep 6;146(10):e141

[14] Aboyans V, Bjo M, Germany SD, Espinola-klein C, France SK, Poland MT. 2017 ESC guidelines on the diagnosis and treatment of peripheral arterial diseases, in collaboration with the European society for vascular surgery (ESVS). European Heart Journal. 2018;**39**(9):763-816

[15] Sirimarco G, Amarenco P, Labreuche J, Touboul PJ, Alberts M, Goto S, et al. Carotid atherosclerosis and risk of subsequent coronary event in outpatients with atherothrombosis. Stroke. 2013;**44**(2):373-379

[16] Alekyan BG, Pokrovsky AV, Karapetyan NG, Revishvili AS. A multidisciplinary approach in determining of the prevalence of coronary artery disease and treatment strategies in patients with pathology of the aorta and peripheral arteries. Russian Cardiologic Journal. 2019;(8):8-16

[17] Yadav JS, Wholey MH, Kuntz RE, Fayad P, Katzen BT, Mishkel GJ, et al. Stenting and angioplasty with protection in patients at high risk for endarterectomy investigators. Protected carotid-artery stenting versus endarterectomy in high-risk patients. The New England Journal of Medicine. 2004;**351**(15):1493-1501. DOI: 10.1056/NEJMoa040127

[18] Alekyan BG, Pokrovsky AV, Zotikov AE, Karapetyan NG, Chupin AV, Popov VA, et al. Results of different treatment strateges the patients with combined coronary and carotid artery disease. Endovascular Surgery. 2021;**8**(2):144-153

[19] Goranov G, Nikolov P, Tokmakova M. Revascularization methods in patients with carotid stenosis and concomitant coronary heart disease. Folia Med (Plovdiv). 2023;**65**(1):7-15. DOI: 10.3897/folmed.65.e69913

[20] Gluck T. Die modernechirurgie des circulations apparates. BerlKlin. 1898;**129**:1-29

[21] Hirsch AT, Haskal ZJ, Hertzer NR, et al. ACC/AHA 2005 practice guidelines for the management of patients with peripheral arterial disease (lower extremity, renal, mesenteric, and abdominal aortic). Circulation. 2006;**113**(11):e463-e654

[22] Fowkes FG. The measurement of atherosclerotic peripheral arterial disease in epidemiological surveys. International Journal of Epidemiology. 1988;**17**(2):248-254

[23] Fowkes FG, Housley E, Cawood E. Edinburgh artery study: Prevalence of asymptomatic and symptomatic peripheral arterial disease in the general population. International Journal of Epidemiology. 1991;**20**(2):384-392

[24] Savji N, Rockman CB, Skolnick AH, et al. Association between advanced age and vascular disease in different arterial territories: A population database of over 3.6 million subjects. Journal of the American College of Cardiology. 2013;**61**(16):1736-1743

[25] Kullo IJ, Rooke TW. Peripheral artery disease. New England Journal of Medicine. 2016;**374**(9):861-871

[26] Steg PG, Bhatt DL, Wilson PW, et al. One-year cardiovascular event rates

in outpatients with atherothrombosis. JAMA - Journal of the American Medical Association. 2007;**297**(11):1197-1206

[27] Zheng Z-J, Richey Sharrett A, Chambless LE. Associations of ankle-brachial index with clinical coronary heart disease, stroke and preclinical carotid and popliteal atherosclerosis: The atherosclerosis risk in communities (ARIC) study. Atherosclerosis. 1997;**131**:115-125

[28] Fowkes GRF, Rudan D, Rudan I. Comparison of global estimates of prevalence and risk factors for peripheral artery disease in 2000 and 2010: A systematic review and analysis. The Lancet. 2013;**382**(9901):1329-1340

[29] Cacoub P, Cambou JP, Kownator S, et al. Prevalence of peripheral arterial disease in high-risk patients using ankle-brachial index in general practice: A cross-sectional study. International Journal of Clinical Practice. 2009;**63**(1):63-70

[30] Criqui MH, Aboyans V. Epidemiology of peripheral artery disease. Circulation Research. 2015;**116**(9):1509-1526

[31] American Medical Association. Ankle brachial index combined with framingham risk score to predict cardiovascular events and mortality a meta-analysis/American medical association. JAMA - Journal of the American Medical Association. 2008;**300**(2):197-208

[32] Conte MS, Pomposelli FB, Clair DG, et al. Society for vascular surgery practice guidelines for atherosclerotic occlusive disease of the lower extremities: Management of asymptomatic disease and claudication. Journal of Vascular Surgery. 2015;**61**(3):2S-41S.e1

[33] Mcfalls EO, Ward HB, Moritz TE, et al. Coronary-artery revascularization before elective major vascular surgery. New England Journal of Medicine. 2004;**351**(27):2795-2804

[34] Landesberg G, Mosseri M. PRO: Preoperative coronary revascularization in high-risk patients undergoing vascular surgery. Anesthesia and Analgesia. 2008;**106**(3):759-763

[35] Raghunathan A, Rapp JH, Littooy F, et al. Postoperative outcomes for patients undergoing elective revascularization for critical limb ischemia and intermittent claudication: A subanalysis of the coronary artery revascularization prophylaxis (CARP) trial. Journal of Vascular Surgery. 2006;**43**(6):1175-1182

[36] Monaco M, Stassano P, Tommaso D. Systematic strategy of prophylactic coronary angiography improves long-term outcome after major vascular surgery in medium- to high-risk patients. A prospective, randomized study. Journal of the American College of Cardiology. 2009;**54**(11):989-996

[37] Bailey SR, Beckman JA, Dao Bailey SR. ACC/AHA/SCAI/SIR/SVM 2018 appropriate use criteria for peripheral artery intervention: A report of the American College of Cardiology appropriate use criteria task force, American Heart Association, society for cardiovascular angiography and interventions. Journal of the American College of Cardiology. 2019;**73**(2):214-237

[38] Cho W, Kim G, Kim H. Prediction of coronary artery disease in patients with lower extremity peripheral artery disease. International Heart Journal. 2015;**56**(2):209-212

[39] Shu J, Santulli G. Update on peripheral artery disease:

Epidemiology and evidence-based facts. Atherosclerosis. 2018;**275**:379-381

[40] Eskelinen E, Lepäntalo M, Hietala EM. Lower limb amputations in Southern Finland in 2000 and trends up to 2001. European Journal of Vascular and Endovascular Surgery. 2004;**27**(2):193-200

[41] Thejasvi T, Caitlin K, Ehrin T. Peripheral artery disease in patients with diabetes: Epidemiology, mechanisms, and outcomes. World Journal of Diabetes. 2015;**6**(7):961

[42] Grundy S, Pasternak R, Greenland P. Assessment of cardiovascular risk by use of multiple-risk-factor assessment equations. Circulation. 1999;**100**(13):1481-1492

[43] Her K, Choi W, Park W. Concomitant peripheral artery disease and asymptomatic coronary artery disease: A management strategy. Annals of Vascular Surgery. 2008;**22**(5):649-656

[44] Hur D, Kizilgul M, Aung W. Frequency of coronary artery disease in patients undergoing peripheral artery disease surgery. American Journal of Cardiology. 2012;**110**(5):736-740

[45] Duran N, Duran I, Gürel E. Coronary artery disease in patients with peripheral artery disease. Heart and Lung: Journal of Acute and Critical Care. 2010;**39**(2):116-120

[46] Norgren L, Hiatt W, Dormandy J. Inter-society consensus for the management of peripheral arterial disease (TASC II). Journal of Vascular Surgery. 2007;**45**(1):5-67

[47] Klimontov VV. Impact of glycemic variability on cardiovascular risk in diabetes. Cardiology. 2018;**58**(10):80-87

[48] Kolh P, Wijns W, Danchin N, Di Mario C, Falk V, Folliguet T, et al. Guidelines on myocardial revascularization. European Journal of Cardio-Thoracic Surgery. 2010;**38**:S1-S52

[49] Reinecke H, Unrath M, Freisinger E. Peripheral arterial disease and critical limb ischaemia: Still poor outcomes and lack of guideline adherence. European Heart Journal. 2015;**36**(15):932-938

[50] Agnelli G, Cimminiello C, Meneghetti G. Low ankle-brachial index predicts an adverse 1-year outcome after acute coronary and cerebrovascular events. Journal of Thrombosis and Haemostasis. 2006;**4**(12):2599-2606

[51] Brevetti G, Piscione F, Silvestro A. Increased inflammatory status and higher prevalence of three-vessel coronary artery disease in patients with concomitant coronary and peripheral atherosclerosis. Thrombosis and Haemostasis. 2003;**89**:1058-1063

[52] Ohman M, Bhatt D, Steg G. The reduction of atherothrombosis for continued health (REACH) registry: An international, prospective, observational investigation in subjects at risk for atherothrombotic events-study design. American Heart Journal. 2006;**151**(4):786-789

[53] Chen C, Singh D, Armstrong J. Long-term comparative outcomes of patients with peripheral artery disease with and without concomitant coronary artery disease. American Journal of Cardiology. 2017;**119**(8):1146-1152

[54] Nishijima A, Yamamoto N, Yoshida R. Coronary artery disease in patients with critical limb ischemia undergoing major amputation or not. Plastic and Reconstructive Surgery - Global Open. 2017;**5**:1-4

[55] Soga Y, Iida O, Takahaera M. Two-year life expectancy in patients with critical limb ischemia. JACC: Cardiovascular Interventions. 2014;7(12):1444-1449

[56] Hertzer N, Beven E, Young J. Coronary artery disease in peripheral vascular patients. Annals of Surgery. 1984;**199**(2):223-233

[57] Alekyan BG, Pokrovskiy AV, Karapetyan NG, Chupin AV, Varava AB, Mitish VA, et al. Immediate results of endovascular treatment of patients with combined lesion of coronary arteries and critical lower limb ischemia. Endovascular Surgery. 2020;**7**(1):24-33

[58] Lee M, Rha S, Han S. Clinical outcomes of patients with critical limb ischemia who undergo routine coronary angiography and subsequent percutaneous coronary intervention. The Journal of Invasive Cardiology. 2015;**27**(4):213-217

[59] Neumann F, Sechtem U, Banning A. 2019 ESC guidelines for the diagnosis and management of chronic coronary syndromes. European Heart Journal. 2020;**41**(3):407-477

[60] Kertai M. Preoperative coronary revascularization in high-risk patients undergoing vascular surgery: A core review. Anesthesia and Analgesia. 2008;**106**(3):751-758

[61] Davies G. Criticial limb ischemia: Epidemiology. Methodist DeBakey Cardiovascular Journal. 2012;**8**(4):10-14

[62] Jude E, Oyibo S, Chalmers N. Peripheral arterial disease in diabetic and nondiabetic patients. Diabetes Care. 2001;**24**(8):1433-1437

[63] Wojtasik-Bakalarz J, Ruzsa Z, Rakowski T. Impact of coronary artery disease and diabetes mellitus on the long-term follow-up in patients after retrograde recanalization of the femoropopliteal arterial region. Journal of Diabetes Research. 2019;**2019**:6

[64] Jämsén T, Manninen H, Tulla H. Infrainguinal revascularization because of claudication: Total long-term outcome of endovascular and surgical treatment. Journal of Vascular Surgery. 2003;**37**(4):808-815

[65] Shammas N. Epidemiology, classification, and modifiable risk factors of peripheral arterial disease. Vascular Health and Risk Management. 2007;**3**(2):229-234

[66] Kesson EM, Allardice GM, George WD, Burns HJ, Morrison DS. Effects of multidisciplinary team working on breast cancer survival: Retrospective, comparative, interventional cohort study of 13 722 women. BMJ. 2012;**344**:e2718

[67] Ray-Coquard I, Thiesse P, Ranchere-Vince D, Chauvin F, Bobin JY, Sunyach MP, et al. Conformity to clinical practice guidelines, multidisciplinary management and outcome of treatment for soft tissue sarcomas. Annals of Oncology. 2004;**15**:307-315

[68] Kristensen SD, Knuuti J, Saraste A, Anker S, Bøtker HE, et al. 2014 ESC/ESA guidelines on non-cardiac surgery: Cardiovascular assessment and management: The joint task force on non-cardiac surgery: Cardiovascular assessment and management of the European society of cardiology (ESC) and the European society of anaesthesiology (ESA). European Heart Journal. 2014;**35**(35):2383-2431

[69] Aboyans V, Ricco JB, Bartelink MLE, Björck M, Brodmann M, Cohnert T, et al. 2017 ESC guidelines on the diagnosis and

treatment of peripheral arterial diseases, in collaboration with the European Society for vascular surgery (ESVS) document covering atherosclerotic disease of extracranial carotid and vertebral, mesenteric, renal, upper and lower extremity arteries endorsed by: The European stroke organization (ESO) the task force for the diagnosis and treatment of peripheral arterial diseases of the European Society of Cardiology (ESC) and of the European Society for Vascular. European Heart Journal. 2017;**39**(9):763-816

[70] Patel MR, Dai D, Hernandez AF, Douglas PS, Messenger J, Garratt KN, et al. Prevalence and predictors of nonobstructive coronary artery disease identified with coronary angiography in contemporary clinical practice. American Heart Journal. 2014;**167**(6):846-852

Chapter 2

Perioperative Use of Impella 5.0/5.5 in High-Risk Coronary Artery Bypass Grafting

Takashi Murashita

Abstract

Coronary artery bypass grafting in patients with low ejection fraction is a high-risk operation because of high incidence of postoperative low cardiac output syndrome. Impella 5.0/5.5 is a surgically implanted left ventricular assist device that can unload the left ventricle. It is capable of full circulatory support. A perioperative use of Impella 5.0/5.5 can potentially improve the surgical outcomes of high-risk coronary artery bypass grafting by avoiding postoperative low cardiac output syndrome. However, the outcomes of Impella 5.0/5.5-supported coronary artery bypass grafting have not been reported frequently. In this chapter, the most recent evidence and the pros and cons of the Impella 5.0/5.5 use at the time of high-risk coronary artery bypass grafting are discussed.

Keywords: Impella 5.0/5.5, high-risk coronary artery bypass grafting, low cardiac output syndrome, surgical outcomes, cardiac physiology

1. Introduction

Coronary artery bypass grafting for patients with severely reduced cardiac function is challenging because of the high incidence of postoperative low cardiac output syndrome [1]. A study that investigated 55,515 patients in New York State database reported that patients with low ejection fraction had >4 times higher mortality than patients with high ejection fraction [2].

Low cardiac output syndrome is defined by an inadequate cardiac pump function resulting in impaired oxygen delivery and tissue hypoxia. The incidence of postoperative low cardiac output syndrome has been reported to be 2–27%, and it carries high hospital mortality of 25–50% [3–6]. Preoperative systolic heart failure, especially left ventricular ejection fraction less than 30%, is known to be a major risk factor for postoperative low cardiac output syndrome.

Since the occurrence of low cardiac output syndrome is associated with other morbidities such as renal and pulmonary failure, stroke, myocardial infarction, sepsis, and prolonged hospital stay, it would increase the health care costs. A study that reviewed 59,810 patients having cardiac surgery from 164 hospitals in the United

States showed that hospital costs elevated to $64,041 in patients with low cardiac output syndrome versus $48,086 in patients without the same [4].

Therefore, it is crucial for healthcare providers to understand how to avoid and manage postoperative low cardiac output syndrome after a high-risk coronary artery bypass grafting.

2. Mechanical circulatory support for low cardiac output syndrome

In the setting of postoperative low cardiac output syndrome, there has been an overall increase in the use of temporary mechanical circulatory support.

Intra-aortic balloon pump has been widely used for postoperative circulatory support in patients with reduced cardiac function [7, 8]. However, it usually requires bed rest, which adversely affects patients' recovery and mobility. In addition, intra-aortic balloon pump may not provide adequate circulatory support for a profound cardiogenic shock.

Impella 2.5 and Impella CP have been widely used in the field of percutaneous coronary intervention. They can be percutaneously inserted through the femoral artery or axillary artery. The benefit of prophylactic use of Impella 2.5 or CP in high-risk percutaneous coronary interventions was reported in several studies [9–12]; however, prophylactic use of Impella in high-risk cardiac surgery has been scarcely reported.

Veno-arterial extracorporeal membrane oxygenation is the most advanced mechanical circulatory support device; however, it is associated with high incidence of complications, such as bleeding, thrombosis, vascular complications, acute renal failure, stroke, and infections. Another disadvantage includes patient immobility.

3. Introduction of Impella 5.0/5.5

Impella 5.0/5.5 with SmartAssist (Abiomed, Danvers, Massachusetts, United States of America) is a surgically implanted heart pump that unloads the left ventricle and therefore can reduce ventricular work. It is composed of 19 Fr microaxial pump and 21 Fr cannula mounted on a 9 Fr drive-line/bearing purge delivery catheter (**Figure 1**). The tip of the Impella is equipped with optical sensor technology, which can be detected by echocardiography so that the proper positioning of the device can be facilitated.

Impella 5.5 is capable of full circulatory support, delivering up to 6.2 L/min. The indication of Impella 5.5 is short-term (14 days) use for the treatment of ongoing cardiogenic shock that occurs immediately (< 48 hours) following acute myocardial infarction or open-heart surgery or in the setting of cardiomyopathy, including peripartum cardiomyopathy, or myocarditis as a result of isolated left ventricular failure that is not responsive to optimal medical management and conventional treatment measures (including volume loading and use of vasopressors and inotropes, with or without intra-aortic balloon pump). The use of Impella 5.5 was approved by the Food and Drug Administration in 2019, and since then, more than 10,000 implants have been performed. In recent years, Impella 5.0/5.5 has been used as a perioperative hemodynamic support at the time of high-risk cardiac surgery. In addition to providing the adequate circulatory support, Impella 5.0/5.5 enables patients to ambulate, and it could optimize recovery.

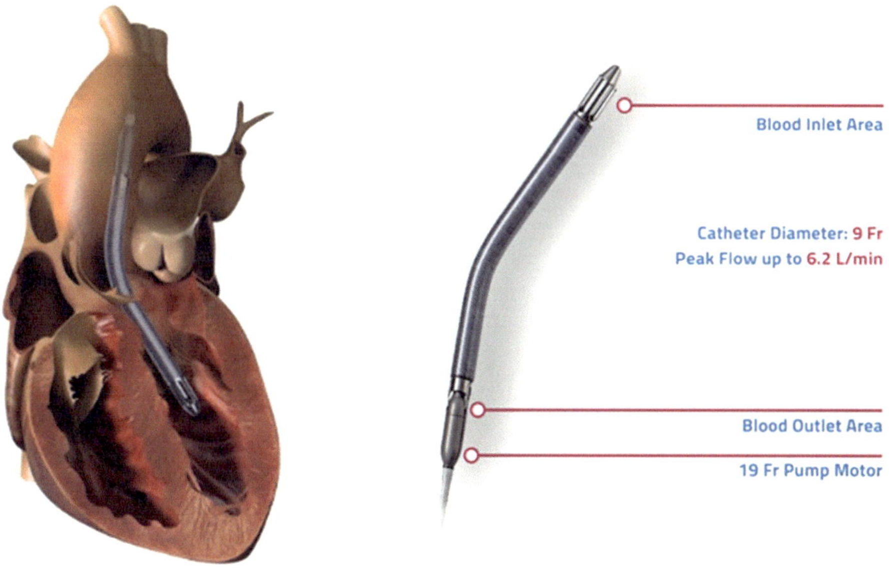

Figure 1.
A scheme of Impella 5.5.

A first multicenter prospective study of Impella 5/0/LD for patients developing cardiogenic shock or low cardiac output syndrome after weaning of cardiopulmonary bypass (RECOVER I) was reported in 2013 [13]. Sixteen patients were enrolled; all patients provided informed consent. The Impella 5.0/LD was inserted *via* the femoral artery or directly to the ascending aorta. The mean preoperative ejection fraction was 23+/−7%, and the patients had multiple comorbidities with high predicted risk of mortality. Despite that, the surgical outcomes were very good; 30-day, 6-month, and 1-year survival was 94, 81, and 75%, respectively.

4. Physiologic change after Impella placement

The most important physiologic effect of Impella is unloading the left ventricle, reducing left ventricular end diastolic pressure and left ventricular wall tension, and consequently decreasing left ventricular work and myocardial oxygen demand.

Secondary, Impella could result in an increase in mean arterial pressure, diastolic pressure, cardiac output, and consequently cardiac power output (calculated by mean arterial pressure x cardiac output/451). It could improve coronary perfusion and systemic perfusion.

Third, Impella could decrease pulmonary capillary pressure and reduce the right ventricular afterload.

The automated Impella Controller displays a real-time hemodynamic and catheter position information (**Figure 2**). This includes the mean arterial pressure, a left ventricular end diastolic pressure, total cardiac output, native cardiac output, and cardiac power output. These numbers can be utilized for patient management and during the weaning process. The Impella Controller can be accessible from any internet-connected device.

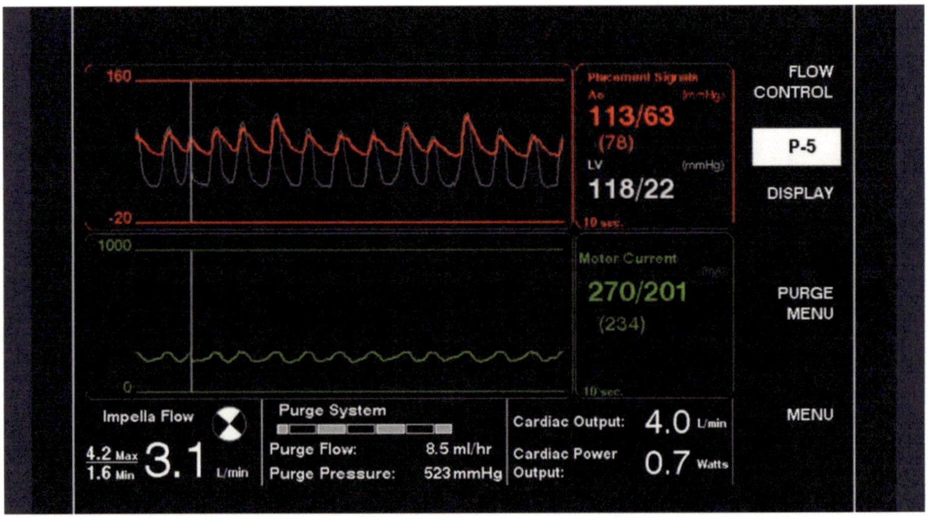

Figure 2.
Automated Impella controlled home screen.

Impella technology is load-dependent but not rhythm-dependent like intra-aortic balloon pump, which leads to a number of physiologic implications. The flow of Impella is afterload-sensitive in that forward flow through the pump decreases with increasing ventriculo-aortic pressure gradient. This sensitivity accounts for the characteristic phasic motor current fluctuations during the cardiac cycle with the highest pump flow and motor current achieved during systole when the gradient between left ventricle and aorta is minimal. This characteristic phasic flow pattern is reported as maximum and minimum flows on the Automated Impella Controller. The phasic motor current is also used in the positioning monitoring algorithm and allows for precise flow calculation. Furthermore, pump flow is preload-dependent because the pump needs sufficient inflow for normal pump output. In patients with acute hemodynamic distress due to left ventricular failure, preload is normally sufficient for normal pump action. Yet extremely impaired inflow may be observed in situations where left ventricular filling pressure is low, the left ventricular cavity is small, or severe right ventricular function impairment is present [14].

5. Implantation technique of Impella 5.0/5.5

The Impella 5.0/5.5 can be implanted *via* the axillary or subclavian artery [15], innominate artery [16, 17], and the ascending aorta (**Figure 3**) [18–20]. Since sternotomy is usually performed at the time of coronary artery bypass grafting, our favorite approach is through the ascending aorta. One of the advantages of the ascending aorta route is the nonnecessity of intraoperative fluoroscopy, which is usually required in the axillary or subclavian artery insertion.

The indications for use of Impella 5.0/5.5 are (a) severe left ventricular dysfunction (left ventricular ejection fraction <30%); (b) estimated prolonged use of cardiopulmonary bypass; (c) comorbidities such as liver disease, chronic kidney disease, chronic obstructive pulmonary disease, and peripheral vascular disease; (d) poor-quality targets, and a combination of these. The contraindications for use of Impella

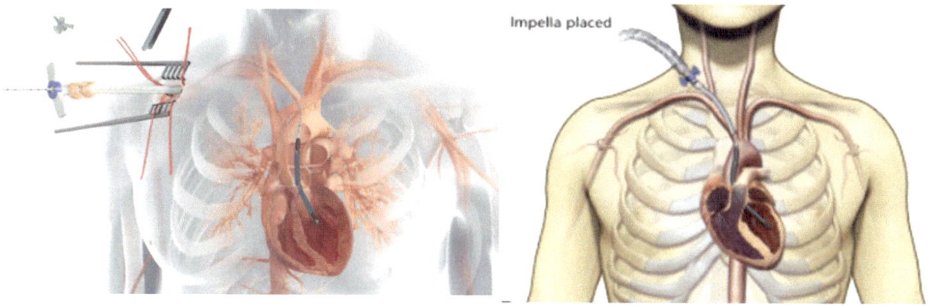

Figure 3.
A scheme of Impella 5.5 insertion via the right axillary artery (left) and innominate artery (right).

5.0/5.5 are (a) mechanical aortic valve prosthesis, (b) aortic valve stenosis (equivalent to an orifice area of 0.6 cm^2 or less), (c) moderate to severe aortic insufficiency, (d) severe right heart failure, (e) combined cardiorespiratory failure, and (f) left ventricular thrombus.

We prefer to place Impella 5.5 prophylactically in high-risk cases, rather than placing it emergently after failing to wean cardiopulmonary bypass.

Our technique for Impella 5.5 placement *via* the ascending aorta is (a) initiation of the cardiopulmonary bypass with a distal ascending aorta cannulation; (b) a partial aortic clamp on the ascending aorta and aortotomy with adequate length; (c) a beveled 10-mm graft anastomosis to the ascending aorta in a side-to-end fashion at least 7 cm above the aortic valve; (d) a small incision is made in the left neck, and the 10 mm graft is tunneled above the skin; (e) aortic cross clamp and completion of coronary artery bypass grafting as usual; (f) insertion of Impella sheath through the 10-mm graft; (g) advancement of J-wire and pig-tail catheter into the left ventricle under a transesophageal echo guidance; (h) advancement of Impella guidewire into the left ventricle under a transesophageal echo guidance; (i) advancement of Impella 5.5 pump through the guidewire, the tip of Impella should be placed about 5 cm below the aortic valve and it should point toward the cardiac apex and away from the septal

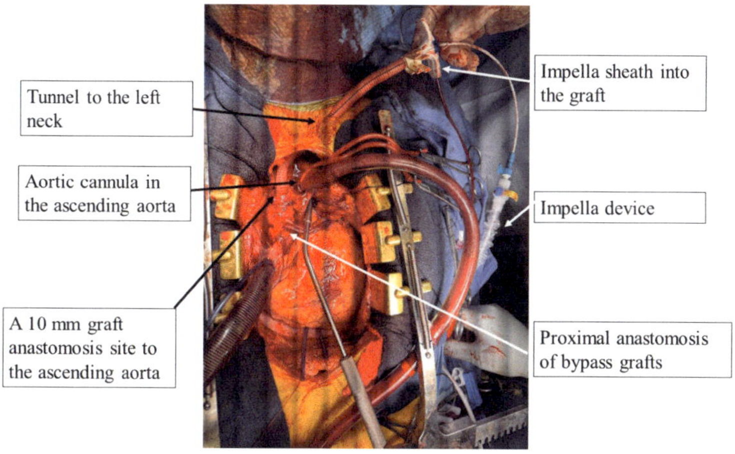

Figure 4.
An intraoperative picture of Impella 5.5 insertion into the ascending aorta via a prosthetic graft.

wall and mitral valve; (j) initiation of Impella 5.5 device; (h) removal of the Impella sheath and trim the graft to the neck incision; and (i) weaning of cardiopulmonary bypass and chest closure. The intraoperative picture is shown in **Figure 4**.

The tips and tricks for this technique are (a) make an adequate length of aortotomy, (b) bevel the graft so that anastomosis can be bigger than the circle area of 10-mm graft, (c) a transesophageal echo guidance (fluoroscopy is not usually necessary), (d) manual manipulation can be used when the Impella pump is passed through the graft anastomosis site, (e) the advancement of Impella could be easier if the blood is returned to the patient from the cardiopulmonary bypass circuit, and (f) do not make the graft length too short, because that would make the future Impella removal difficult.

6. Perioperative management of Impella 5.0/5.5

After the insertion of the Impella, the position of the device should be confirmed routinely with at least two views of transthoracic echocardiography such as parasternal long axis and apical four chamber views. Impella 5.5 does not have a pigtail in the tip as opposed to Impella 5.0. The malposition of the device could easily happen. The device could attach or push the ventricular septum if it is rotated away from the mitral valve and that could cause suction events. The Impella pump needs to be away from the ventricular septal wall. Functional mitral stenosis caused by the dislocation of the device shaft on the anterior mitral leaflet was reported [21]. A big benefit of Impella system through the direct aorta approach is that patients can be extubated and are able to ambulate with Impella system. That can promote patients' quick recovery.

Balthazar and colleagues reviewed the management of mechanical circulatory support [22]. The weaning of Impella should be managed by a multidisciplinary team including cardiac surgeons, cardiologists, intensivists, and perfusionists. Before starting weaning, the patients should have normal lactated levels and on low pressors or inotropes. A daily turndown of the Impella flow with a cautious hemodynamic evaluation should be attempted. When the increase in native cardiac output after weaning of Impella meets the patients' metabolic needs and does not result in significant increases in ventricular pressures, Impella could be removed.

The removal of Impella 5.0/5.5 can be done even with local anesthesia in the intensive care unit. No repeat sternotomy is required. After the Impella is weaned off, the device is pulled out from the graft. The graft is clamped and tied off with heavy silk string or oversewn with monofilament polypropylene sutures. The graft can be closed with surgical staplers. The stump of the graft is put back into the neck incision, and the incision is closed.

7. Postoperative outcomes

The postoperative outcomes of coronary artery bypass grafting with a support of Impella 5.0/5.5 have not been reported frequently. The postoperative outcomes of Impella supported CABG are summarized in **Table 1**. Overall, the reported outcomes have been excellent in consideration of high-risk patients' population.

	Number of cases	Operation	30-day mortality	Duration of Impella
Benke et al. [23]	14	10 coronary artery bypass grafting, 2 aortic valve surgery, and 2 coronary artery bypass grafting and valvular surgery	7.2%	4 days
Ranganath et al. [24]	13	All coronary artery bypass grafting	0%	5.7 days
Sabra et al. [25]	9	5 isolated coronary artery bypass grafting, 4 coronary artery bypass grafting, and valvular surgery	11%	Not reported
Akay et al. [26]	1	Off-pump coronary artery bypass grafting	100%	2 days
Tavilla et al. [27]	1	Off-pump coronary artery bypass grafting	0%	Not reported
Smith et al. [28]	4	All coronary artery bypass grafting	25%	0–500 hours
Ramzy et al. [29]	12	7 postcardiotomy cardiogenic shock, 5 coronary artery bypass grafting	16.4%	Not reported
Funamoto et al. [30]	12	7 isolated coronary artery bypass grafting, and 5 valve or combined valve/coronary/aortic procedure	0%	6.3 days
Marin-Cuartas et al. [31]	19	Postcardiotomy cardiogenic shock	15.8%	Not reported

Table 1.
Surgical outcomes of Impella-supported coronary artery bypass grafting.

8. Complications of Impella 5.0/5.5 use

There are some complications that are specifically related to Impella 5.0/5.5 use. Ghannam and colleagues reported a case of aortic valve injury related to the Impella 5.5 use [32]. The Impella 5.5 was removed on postoperative day 8, and the patient went into cardiogenic shock due to aortic valve leaflet injury, which required aortic valve replacement.

Pump thrombosis is a rare complication, but it has been reported [33]. Systemic anticoagulation with heparin is suggested; however, it can increase the risk of bleeding [34, 35]. Currently, there are no clear data in terms of optimal anticoagulation regimen [36].

Left ventricular perforation could also happen because of the manipulation of the guidewire and cannula into the left ventricle. There were multiple case reports for that [37–41]. Surgeons should suspect left ventricular perforation when there is a newly discovered pericardial effusion, change in waveform on the Impella controller placement signal, or patients' rapid deterioration.

Debenham and colleagues reported adverse events related to Impella 5.0/5.5 in the American College of Cardiology meeting, using the manufacturer and user facility device experience database (the abstract is available at https://www.jacc.org/doi/epdf/10.1016/S0735-1097%2822%2901478-4). Compared with Impella 5.0, the Impella 5.5 had a higher incidence of pump stoppage (51.7% vs. 10.9%, $p < 0.001$) and LV perforation (13.3% vs. 1.7%, $p < 0.001$) with a lower incidence of stroke (0% vs.

8.4%, $p < 0.021$), mitral valve regurgitation (1.6% vs. 11.8%, $p < 0.02$), hemorrhage (8.3% vs. 21.8%, $p < 0.024$), and sepsis (0% vs. 6.7%, $p < 0.04$). There was no difference in the incidence of vascular injury, limb ischemia, aortic valve damage, pump thrombosis, or hemolysis between the two devices.

The other complications include bleeding, infection, stroke, and acute kidney injury, which are accompanied with usual coronary artery bypass grafting. Since the patient population is sicker than regular patients, the occurrence of complications was reported to be higher than normal.

9. Conclusions

The Impella 5.0/5.5 can be easily inserted into the ascending aorta *via* a prosthetic graft and can provide a tremendous hemodynamic support during and after high-risk coronary artery bypass grafting. It could improve surgical outcomes by avoiding a postoperative low cardiac output syndrome, which is associated with high operative mortality. Direct insertion of an Impella 5.0/5.5 to the ascending aorta allows the patients to ambulate and recover until heart function improves. The explanation of the device is easy and does not require a repeat sternotomy.

Author details

Takashi Murashita
Clinical Surgery, Division of Cardiothoracic Surgery, Department of Surgery, University of Missouri, Columbia, Missouri, USA

*Address all correspondence to: tmurashita@gmail.com; murashitat@health.missouri.edu

References

[1] Kochar A, Zheng Y, van Diepen S, Mehta RH, Westerhout CM, Mazer DC, et al. Predictors and associated clinical outcomes of low cardiac output syndrome following cardiac surgery: Insights from the LEVO-CTS trial. European Heart Journal Acute Cardiovascular Care. 2022;**11**(11):818-825. DOI: 10.1093/ehjacc/zuac114

[2] Topkara VK, Cheema FH, Kesavaramanujam S, Mercando ML, Cheema AF, Namerow PB, et al. Coronary artery bypass grafting in patients with low ejection fraction. Circulation. 2005;**112**(9 Suppl):I344-I350. DOI: 10.1161/CIRCULATIONAHA.104.526277

[3] Algarni KD, Maganti M, Yau TM. Predictors of low cardiac output syndrome after isolated coronary artery bypass surgery: Trends over 20 years. The Annals of Thoracic Surgery. 2011;**92**(5):1678-1684. DOI: 10.1016/j.athoracsur.2011.06.017. Epub 2011 September 21

[4] Duncan AE, Kartashov A, Robinson SB, Randall D, Zhang K, Luber J, et al. Risk factors, resource use, and cost of postoperative low cardiac output syndrome. The Journal of Thoracic and Cardiovascular Surgery. 2022;**163**(5):1890-1898.e10. DOI: 10.1016/j.jtcvs.2020.06.125. Epub 2020 July 16

[5] Ding W, Ji Q, Shi Y, Ma R. Predictors of low cardiac output syndrome after isolated coronary artery bypass grafting. International Heart Journal. 2015;**56**(2):144-149. DOI: 10.1536/ihj.14-231. Epub 2015 February 23

[6] Sá MP, Nogueira JR, Ferraz PE, Figueiredo OJ, Cavalcante WC, Cavalcante TC, et al. Risk factors for low cardiac output syndrome after coronary artery bypass grafting surgery. Revista Brasileira de Cirurgia Cardiovascular. 2012;**27**(2):217-223. DOI: 10.5935/1678-9741.20120037

[7] Deppe AC, Weber C, Liakopoulos OJ, Zeriouh M, Slottosch I, Scherner M, et al. Preoperative intra-aortic balloon pump use in high-risk patients prior to coronary artery bypass graft surgery decreases the risk for morbidity and mortality-A meta-analysis of 9,212 patients. Journal of Cardiac Surgery. 2017;**32**(3):177-185. DOI: 10.1111/jocs.13114

[8] Baskett RJ, O'Connor GT, Hirsch GM, Ghali WA, Sabadosa K, Morton JR, et al.; Northern New England Cardiovascular Disease Study Group. A multicenter comparison of intraaortic balloon pump utilization in isolated coronary artery bypass graft surgery. The Annals of Thoracic Surgery. 2003;**76**(6):1988-1992; discussion 1992. DOI: 10.1016/s0003-4975(03)01197-4

[9] van den Buijs DMF, van den Brink FS, Wilgenhof A, Zivelonghi C, Verouden N, Knaapen P, et al. Complex high-risk indicated percutaneous coronary intervention with prophylactic use of the Impella CP ventricular assist device. The Journal of Invasive Cardiology. 2022;**34**(9):E665-E671. Epub 2022 August 19

[10] Alasnag MA, Gardi DO, Elder M, Kannam H, Ali F, Petrina M, et al. Use of the Impella 2.5 for prophylactic circulatory support during elective high-risk percutaneous coronary intervention. Cardiovascular Revascularization Medicine. 2011;**12**(5):299-303. DOI: 10.1016/j.carrev.2011.02.002. Epub 2011 March 30

[11] Baumann S, Werner N, Ibrahim K, Westenfeld R, Al-Rashid F, Sinning JM, et al. Indication and short-term clinical outcomes of high-risk percutaneous coronary intervention with microaxial Impella® pump: Results from the German Impella® registry. Clinical Research in Cardiology. 2018;**107**(8):653-657. DOI: 10.1007/s00392-018-1230-6. Epub 2018 March 8

[12] Iliodromitis KE, Kahlert P, Plicht B, Hoffmann AC, Eggebrecht H, Erbel R, et al. High-risk PCI in acute coronary syndromes with Impella LP 2.5 device support. International Journal of Cardiology. 2011;**153**(1):59-63. DOI: 10.1016/j.ijcard.2010.08.039. Epub 2010 September 9

[13] Griffith BP, Anderson MB, Samuels LE, Pae WE Jr, Naka Y, Frazier OH. The RECOVER I: A multicenter prospective study of Impella 5.0/LD for postcardiotomy circulatory support. The Journal of Thoracic and Cardiovascular Surgery. 2013;**145**(2):548-554. DOI: 10.1016/j.jtcvs.2012.01.067. Epub 2012 March 9

[14] Burzotta F, Trani C, Doshi SN, Townend J, van Geuns RJ, Hunziker P, et al. Impella ventricular support in clinical practice: Collaborative viewpoint from a European expert user group. International Journal of Cardiology. 2015;**201**:684-691. DOI: 10.1016/j.ijcard.2015.07.065. Epub 2015 July 30

[15] Schultz J, Duval S, Shaffer A, John R, Alexy T, Martin CM, et al. Axillary or subclavian Impella 5.0 support in cardiogenic shock: A systematic review and meta-analysis. ASAIO Journal. 2022;**68**(2):233-238. DOI: 10.1097/MAT.0000000000001452

[16] Bertolin S, Maj G, Cavozza C, Cardinale A, Pullara A, Audo A, et al. Impella 5.0/5.5 implantation via innominate artery: Further expanding the opportunities for temporary mechanical circulatory support. Journal of Clinical Medicine. 2022;**11**(19):5917. DOI: 10.3390/jcm11195917

[17] Bouhout I, Nguyen SN, Barry OM, Bacha EA, Goldstone AB. Transinnominate Impella 5.5 insertion as a bridge to transplantation in a pediatric patient in refractory cardiogenic shock. JTCVS Techniques. 2022;**14**:201-203. DOI: 10.1016/j.xjtc.2022.06.005. eCollection 2022 August

[18] Anderson M, Smith D, Kane P, Lee R, Khalpey Z, Williams J. Impella 5.5 direct aortic implant and explant techniques. The Annals of Thoracic Surgery. 2021;**111**(5):e373-e375. DOI: 10.1016/j.athoracsur.2020.09.069. Epub 2020 December 17

[19] Salas de Armas IA, Shirafkan A, Akay MH, Patel J, Patel MK, Marcano J, et al. Transaortic placement of percutaneous mechanical support device via partial sternotomy: Feasible option for unsuitable axillary artery access. Innovations (Philadelphia, Pa.). 2022;**17**(5):377-381. DOI: 10.1177/15569845221123535. Epub 2022 October 2

[20] Choi DC, Anderson MB, Batsides GP. Insertion of the Impella 5.0 left ventricular assist device via right anterior mini-thoracotomy: A novel practical approach. Innovations (Philadelphia, Pa.). 2011;**6**(4):265-266. DOI: 10.1097/IMI.0b013e31822b36b8

[21] Toggweiler S, Jamshidi P, Erne P. Functional mitral stenosis: A rare complication of the Impella assist device. European Journal of Echocardiography. 2008;**9**(3):412-413. DOI: 10.1093/ejechocard/jen029. Epub 2008 March 30

[22] Balthazar T, Vandenbriele C, Verbrugge FH, Den Uil C, Engström A, Janssens S, et al. Managing patients with short-term mechanical circulatory support: JACC review topic of the week. Journal of the American College of Cardiology. 2021;**77**(9):1243-1256. DOI: 10.1016/j.jacc.2020.12.054

[23] Benke K, Korça E, Boltjes A, Stengl R, Hofmann B, Matin M, et al. Preventive Impella® support in high-risk patients undergoing cardiac surgery. Journal of Clinical Medicine. 2022;**11**(18):5404. DOI: 10.3390/jcm11185404

[24] Ranganath NK, Nafday HB, Zias E, Hisamoto K, Chen S, Kon ZN, et al. Concomitant temporary mechanical support in high-risk coronary artery bypass surgery. Journal of Cardiac Surgery. 2019;**34**(12):1569-1572. DOI: 10.1111/jocs.14295. Epub 2019 October 26

[25] Sabra MJ, Andrews WG, Crandall ML, Pirris JP. The postoperative use of Impella as a ventricular assist device in high-risk patients undergoing coronary artery bypass surgery: A case series and comparison. Journal of Cardiac Surgery. 2020;**35**(1):113-117. DOI: 10.1111/jocs.14367. Epub 2019 December 3

[26] Akay MH, Frazier OH. Impella recover 5.0 assisted coronary artery bypass grafting. Journal of Cardiac Surgery. 2010;**25**(5):606-607. DOI: 10.1111/j.1540-8191.2010.01071.x

[27] Tavilla G, Beckles DL, Morris P, Reddy RC. Off-pump myocardial revascularization with Impella 5.5-assisted for cardiogenic shock. Journal of Cardiac Surgery. 2021;**36**(10):3898-3900. DOI: 10.1111/jocs.15778. Epub 2021 Junuary 30

[28] Smith NJ, Ramamurthi A, Joyce LD, Durham LA, Kohmoto T, Joyce DL. Temporary mechanical circulatory support prevents the occurrence of a low-output state in high-risk coronary artery bypass grafting: A case series. Journal of Cardiac Surgery. 2021;**36**(3):864-871. DOI: 10.1111/jocs.15309. Epub 2021 January 11

[29] Ramzy D, Soltesz E, Anderson M. New surgical circulatory support system outcomes. ASAIO Journal. 2020;**66**(7):746-752. DOI: 10.1097/MAT.0000000000001194

[30] Funamoto M, Kunavarapu C, Kwan MD, Matsuzaki Y, Shah M, Ono M. Single center experience and early outcomes of Impella 5.5. Frontiers in Cardiovascular Medicine. 2023;**10**:1018203. DOI: 10.3389/fcvm.2023.1018203. eCollection 2023

[31] Marin-Cuartas M, Wehrmann K, Höbartner M, Lehmann S, Etz CD, Saeed D, et al. Perioperative temporary mechanical circulatory support with Impella in cardiac surgery patients. The Journal of Cardiovascular Surgery. 2022;**63**(2):229-236. DOI: 10.23736/S0021-9509.22.12173-7. Epub 2022 February 10

[32] Ghannam AD, Takebe M, Harmon TS, Tatum S, Pirris J. Aortic valve leaflet disruption: A severe complication of Impella 5.5. Cureus. 2021;**13**(2):e13235. DOI: 10.7759/cureus.13235

[33] Ranc S, Sibellas F, Green L. Acute intraventricular thrombosis of an impella LP 5.0 device in an ST-elevated myocardial infarction complicated by cardiogenic shock. The Journal of Invasive Cardiology. 2013;**25**(1):E1-E3

[34] Karami M, den Uil CA, Ouweneel DM, Scholte NT,

Engström AE, Akin S, et al. Mechanical circulatory support in cardiogenic shock from acute myocardial infarction: Impella CP/5.0 versus ECMO. European Heart Journal Acute Cardiovascular Care. 2020;**9**(2):164-172. DOI: 10.1177/2048872619865891. Epub 2019 July 29

[35] Dhruva SS, Ross JS, Mortazavi BJ, Hurley NC, Krumholz HM, Curtis JP, et al. Association of use of an intravascular microaxial left ventricular assist device vs intra-aortic balloon pump with in-hospital mortality and major bleeding among patients with acute myocardial infarction complicated by cardiogenic shock. JAMA. 2020;**323**(8):734-745. DOI: 10.1001/jama.2020.0254

[36] Zaky M, Kawabori M. Anticoagulation strategy, the Achilles' heel while on prolonged Impella 5.5 support. ASAIO Journal. 2023;**69**(6):e285. DOI: 10.1097/MAT.0000000000001908. Epub 2023 March 7

[37] Glazier JJ, Kaki A. Left ventricular perforation after Impella placement. Catheterization and Cardiovascular Interventions. 2018;**92**(4):827. DOI: 10.1002/ccd.27451. Epub 2017 December 27

[38] Peritz DC, Linstroth L, Selzman CH, Gilbert EM. Left ventricular perforation after Impella® placement in a patient with cardiogenic shock. Catheterization and Cardiovascular Interventions. 2018;**91**(5):894-896. DOI: 10.1002/ccd.27329. Epub 2017 September 25

[39] Glazier JJ, Kaki A, Baciewicz F. Successful treatment of left ventricular perforation occurring after insertion of an Impella device. International Journal of Angiology. 2020;**29**(3):202-204. DOI: 10.1055/s-0038-1666971. Epub 2018 July 30

[40] Salas de Armas IA, Kumar S, Almustafa A, Akkanti B, Akay MH, Patel MK, et al. Left ventricular rupture after Impella® placement during high-risk percutaneous coronary intervention. Cardiovascular Revascularization Medicine. 2020;**21**(11S):100-102. DOI: 10.1016/j.carrev.2019.06.011. Epub 2019 January 30

[41] Mizuno A, Kawamoto S, Uda S, Tatsumi K, Takeda C, Tanaka T, et al. A case of left ventricular free wall rupture after insertion of an IMPELLA® left ventricular assist device diagnosed by transesophageal echocardiography. JA Clinical Reports. 2021;**7**(1):38. DOI: 10.1186/s40981-021-00444-w

Chapter 3

Perioperative Ultrasound Flow Evaluation in Grafts and Native Vessel during CABG

Bedrudin Banjanović, Edin Kabil, Nedžad Kadrić, Emir Mujanović, Mirza Dilić, Mehmed Kulić, Samed Djedović, Amel Hadžimegmedagić, Muhamed Djedović, Zina Lazović, Sevleta Avdić, Tarik Selimović, Lejla Divović and Nada Malešić

Abstract

New blood in the vascular bed after coronary artery bypass grafting (CABG) may represent a turning point between ischemia and normal tissue nutrition. Quality control during CABG preoperatively is essential because errors lead to immediate consequences. With an understanding of hemodynamics, we can now search for less invasive tools for quantification of coronary blood flow changes over time after CABG. Ultrasound is becoming a key player for that purpose and we will present its application. Perioperatively, quality control in CABG should include target selection of native coronary arteries, graft selection, anastomose checking, and long-term flow follow-up. Because some grafts are unreachable for ultrasound evaluation, we should examine both arterial venous sides of coronary circulation. We will present the use of classic, epicardial ultrasonography and TTFM probes by looking for stenoses and competitive flow. We will present our research for quantification of new blood in coronary vessels after CABG. There we found constant increase in flow over the early postoperative period (20% per graft). By increasing graft number, coronary flow increases first linearly and then stepwise. Measured data and trends can be used in ambulatory monitoring and screening of ischemic complications after CABG.

Keywords: CABG, quality control, coronary sinus, TTFM, Doppler, LIMA/RIMA, grafts

1. Introduction

Ischemic heart disease (IHD) represents part of cardiovascular disease, which is connected to 30% of deaths worldwide. Especially in low- or moderately-developed countries, where 80% of cardiovascular disease is concentrated. IHD is a disease of coronary arteries and capillary bed that narrows vessel lumen, leading to reduced blood flow below heart needs. Flow reduction during rest is rare except in severely stenotic coronary arteries, hibernated myocardial segments, and after acute myocardial infarction. More often, there is flow reduction during maximal dilatation. The impact of atherosclerotic ischemic heart disease on quality of life and its connection to mortality is well-established.

Three overlapping treatments highly reduce the occurrence of adverse cardiovascular events and are used daily: medication, revascularization by percutaneous intervention, or surgical operation. Complications in macrocirculation during disease progression can be stopped or decelerated with adequate revascularization. ESC guidelines for myocardial revascularization promote the indications for the coronary artery bypass graft (CABG) over percutaneous procedure due to the higher beneficial effects of this procedure. The benefit is especially seen in patients with double vessel disease with proximal left anterior descending (LAD) stenosis, left main disease, triple vessel disease, and some other situations. In our practice and as we know in some other centers even single LAD stenosis is treated surgically if PCI procedure is impossible. When we are dealing with candidates for Re-Do or Re-Re-Do, the indications for surgical revascularization are generally the same as for first surgery. We take into account how big part of myocardium is at risk and the patency of LIMA-LAD ("no LIMA no Case").

As millions of people are in danger to have CVD, 25% will have heart attacks in asymptomatic stage of the disease. All put together suggest that it will be important to develop more accurate method of screening of coronary artery disease and for quality control after revascularization procedures. All revascularization procedures should be subjected to quality control. They can be performed pre-OP, intra-OP, and post-OP. Given the possibility of harvesting of grafts from multiple locations, testing their suitability is necessary and falls under pre-OP quality control. Anatomical and functional tests of native coronary arteries, which are in the domain of the interventional cardiologist during coronary angiography, also fall under PreOP control. Considering the numerous cardiosurgical techniques of CABG OPCAB/ONCAB, graft configurations, and comorbidities, intra-OP quality control is very important and must be systematically carried out during the entire treatment. In the early and late Post-Op period, and due to the processes described in the further part of the text, Post-Op quality control should be carried out primarily to monitor bypass complications (anastomotic stenosis, graft occlusion, competition ...), myocardium, but also possible progression of native coronary disease. As some grafts are inaccessible to flow measurements outside the OR, we also have to take into account their impact on coronary flow. Contemporary and reliable method will be flowmetric measurements on the venous side of the heart (coronary sinus) in addition to all mentioned above.

2. Quality control

CABG quality control is so important that every self-critical cardiac surgeon must always perform it. The reason is that it directly affects the early and late success of the surgical work. Quality control must include not only performed bypasses but also unperformed ones, given that incomplete revascularization is associated with increased mortality. Patency of bypasses is influenced by many variables (surgical technique, local findings, inflow-outflow, experience of the cardiac surgeon, etc.). The above reasons can lead to early anastomotic errors with future graft failure in 1–3%. The percentage is cumulative and increases with the number of anastomoses. Disease progression of native coronary arteries or progression of disease on grafts in the late post-OP period can lead to a decrease in total or regional blood volume in the myocardium. The aforementioned progression may require repeated diagnostic re-evaluation in terms of ischemic heart disease and consequent revascularization (CABG/PCI) and occurs in about 3% [1]. These conditions are much more complex and sometimes, unfortunately, cannot be solved by a cardiac surgeon. That is why early recognition of asymptomatic progression is very important, but it is often delayed, incidental, or discovered after the development of ischemic complications. Therefore, each phase of treatment of ischemic heart disease should be evaluated and documented as much as local personnel and technical possibilities allow. We believe that without going deep into the protocols of cardiac surgery centers, guideliness, experience of cardiac surgeons, the establishment of quality control, and strict adherence can distinguish the Center of Excellence from others. At the same time, it protects us from the law but also from non-benevolent colleagues.

In general, the quality control of CABG requires comprehensive judgment and individualized measures to ensure the safety and long-term outcome of patients. Although the importance of the volume of operations on the outcome and reduction of complications is described in the literature, systematic quality control can sometimes nullify this problem. Namely, Auerbach et al. who analyzed quality control showed that when quality control is maximized, CABG mortality at very low-volume hospitals is similar to very high-volume hospitals. If we transfer the point of this study (detailed and regular quality control of each step) to all other cardiac surgeries, we will probably have significantly better results in smaller centers as well. Of course, we do not want to ignore the connection between volume and experience and results, but we want to emphasize the unused potential of quality control. In this way, we encourage young cardiac surgeons in their professional development.

When to start quality control in surgical myocardial revascularization? The answer is yesterday. Unfortunately, even in centers that are equipped and staffed for detailed perioperative monitoring of bypass effects on coronary flow, these measurements rarely represent the protocol. In general, quality control should be started before the actual operation, and the measurement results should be documented. In this way, the effects of revascularization will be easily monitored during the entire perioperative period.

The analysis should include the anatomy of the target and their functional tests in order to reveal the actual stenoses that will benefit the most from revascularization. Direct ultrasound evaluation of native coronary arteries (LM and RCA) is very difficult and unreliable, so it will not be the subject of this paper. Given that modern ultrasound machines are widely available today, measurement of the venous side of the coronary circulation—flow through the coronary sinus is possible. It gives us additional information about coronary flow, especially since it includes the return of blood from ultrasound-inaccessible grafts (venous bypasses). But, what is important is that the technique used should be simple for ambulatory monitoring. This can only be achieved with non-invasive ultrasound measurements. In addition to the analysis of the flow through the native coronary arteries and coronary sinus, it is necessary to record the anatomy preoperatively and, where possible and necessary, to functionally examine the grafts as well as the circulation that will be left behind after harvesting the grafts. We primarily mean LIMA/RIMA angiography and ultrasound tests of IMAs and Radial artery circulation and VSM/VSP veins. The most common preoperative technique for functional measurement of stenosis of native coronary arteries is—FFR. Functional assessment graft is possible either pre-OP or intra-OP. They include the measurement of flow volume, resistance index, etc. at rest and after drug administration (Adenosine, NTG, Dypiridamol, etc.) and sometimes intra-OP during free flow, which will be discussed later. A good example of a pre-OP analysis of grafts is the radial artery, which should be anatomically evaluated (diameters on ultrasound), and with an ultrasound-enhanced Allen's test to examine its collateral circulation and its potency with an ischemic ultrasound test.

Pre-OP and Post-OP non-invasive assessment of IMA patency is challenging, but duplex ultrasound (DU) can be accepted as a reliable technique. The main goal of the examination is the detection of stenosis/occlusion or flow competition. DU may detect severe (>70%) stenosis by PW Doppler data (peak diastolic velocity/peak systolic velocity < 0.5 and diastolic fraction <50%). Considering that medium-severe stenoses (50–70%) at rest do not show changes in volumetric parameters except for slight accelerations of flow at the stenosis itself, it is possible that they may be missed during imaging. That's why we present the below curve analysis with the use of some form of stress test (adenosine, NTG, Dypiridamol, etc.) in order to reveal borderline stenoses.

Intra-OP quality control includes the use of TTFM, epicardial and classic Doppler probes, and TTE/TEE. The goal is to examine the graft for stenosis, and competition by determining the total flow, flow in the systole/diastole phases, resistance indices, and other characteristics of the flow curve. And to quantify returning blood from coronary sinus, for screening of post-OP follow-up. A conclusion should be made about the potency of grafts, especially composite grafts, expected durability, etc. The best-known and most commonly used quality control tool in OR is the transit time flow measurement (TTFM). TTFM effectively detects the coronary graft failure but often needs additional knowledge to decide the cause of failure. If we add high-resolution epicardial ultrasound to TTFM we can improve the quality, safety, and effectiveness of CABG.

At the end of the day, there are several useful consequences of quality control. Pre-OP we will better choose native target and best graft/graft configuration. Intra-OP we will assess flow and if necessary re-anastomose immediately in OR before severe consequences occur. Post-OP we will detect failing grafts or native vessel stenosis earlier during the follow-up period before complications occur. This is after intra-OP judgment the most important data that we can extract from patient during follow-up. This early detection of failing graft is often challenging, because of technical limitations and because in busy outpatient departments examinations are often performed during rest where there is rest flow, taking into account only basic data from DU. But, even in that situation if we have data about pre-OP quantities of flow (with resistance indexes and other flow curve data analysis), intra-OP flow increase, coronary sinus flow, and expected early increase of flow in post-OP period at least we can individualize trend changes and make some conclusions before severe consequences develop. A typical mentioned situation will be when the graft occludes even without ECG changes, during the early ICU period, while the patient is at bed rest. This is the most important message in this chapter, possibility of noninvasive early detection of failing grafts/native vessels during follow-up. If we are suspicious of the mentioned situation or have a symptomatic patient (with other signs of ischemia) after CABG, there are plenty of diagnostic procedures for case evaluation. We can examine anatomical, functional, and physiological aspects of flow in post-CABG recurrent angina with assessment of left ventricular function, myocardial viability, etc. Furthermore, we can choose the best management strategies for this complex patient population. Who are often older with higher prevalence of comorbidities and complex atherosclerotic lesions. Diagnostic management can include besides re-coronarography other procedure: stress electro and stress echo examination, CT coronarography, MRI, myocardial scintigraphia, PET CT, etc. Some of them have limitations like expenses, radiation exposure, or insufficient sensitivity and specificity. But, in this chapter, we want to focus on pure noninvasive flow detection on the arterial and venous side of coronary circulation.

3. Coronary flow

Normal coronary artery flow is 5% of cardiac output, around 250 ml/min [2]. Resting flow through normal coronary arteries, according to invasive measurements, is 0.5–1.5 ml/gr/min (0.8–1.2 ml/gr/min). At the same time, maximal coronary artery flow is 3–4 ml/gr/min.

Resting flow through severely stenotic coronary arteries (= > 80%), hibernated myocardial segments or infarcted area is <0,5 ml/min/gr. At the same time, maximal coronary artery flow is <1 ml/min/gr.

Resting flow in intermediate stenosis (60–80%) is the same as in healthy coronary arteries but slightly near lower value, with differences in published literature [3]. Maximal flow through intermediate stenosis strongly correlates with degree of stenosis. Flow started to decrease with stenosis of 40% and become same as resting flow in stenosis = > 80%. Patients with microcirculatory disturbances (diabetes, hyperlipoproteinemia, arterial hypertension, nicotine abuse, etc.), even without angiographically evident stenosis also has decreased flow during rest or effort [4]. It is mainly because of vasodilatatory defects of endothelial cells.

After CABG resting net flow increases from 0,65 to 0,78 ml/min/gr and maximal flow increase from 0,85 to 1,0 ml/min/gr. To simplify: there is a 20% increase in blood flow per gram of myocardium for every graft.

CS flow is lower than sum of coronary artery flow. It is because there are: alternative drainage routes (Thebasian veins and tributaries not connected to CS) and because CS drains mainly left coronary artery territory [5]. Severe coronary artery stenosis can decrease the CS blood flow. Revascularization of severely stenotic vessels can increase coronary artery and consequently CS flow. Because of this coronary sinus flow can be used in post-OP Coronary Circulation Assessment by looking at trends over time.

In case we are averaging flow rate over a gram of myocardium (during CS, IMAs, or SVG volumetric measurements) we recommend ASE; Devereux formula for LV mass calculations. Formula is: LVgr = 0,8(1,04(LVDD + PWTD + IVSTD)3-(LVIDD)3)) + 0,6. Here, LVDD is LV diameter in diastole, IVSTD is diastolic diameter of septum, PWTD is diastolic diameter of posterior wall near apex of papillary muscle. With correction of whole myocardium mass by addition of right ventricle mass (according to certain conditions), what is outside of this paper.

4. Recording suites

Regardless of the time of measuring the hemodynamics of the grafts (pre-OP/post-OP), IMA grafts and coronary sinus are always available for measurements. Other grafts (aortocoronary: VSM/VSP or radial artery) are inaccessible to pre-OP/post-OP ultrasound flow measurement techniques. So, intraoperative measurements of all available grafts by DU or TTFM should always be recorded.

4.1 Arterial side of coronary circulation

Preoperative angiographic scan of IMAs is almost always possible and should be "must" in all CABG. Unfortunately, it is not performed routinely. Usually, because of fear of contrast overdose or in emergencies. The left internal mammary artery (LIMA) is the best first choice for performing CABG due to its location and structural characteristics. LIMA arises from the subclavian artery opposite to Thyreocervical trunk. IMAs are bigger in men and on right side [6]. LIMA descends behind the upper six ribs, 1.5 cm from the sternum. LIMA is elastic artery with intima, media, and adventitia layers. The composition of these layers varies throughout the route from the subclavian artery to its epigastric bifurcation. The media layer has two elastic lamina: external (contribution to elastic performance) and internal (contribution to muscular performance). All of these layers account for long patency of the IMAs in CABG surgery. Also, IMAs have fewer endothelial fenestrations and less intercellular junctions, and high intercellular communication. Because of this IMAs are highly resistant to manipulation during harvesting.

4.1.1 Equipment

Early use of Doppler Ultrasonography (DU) for LIMA hemodynamic assessment after CABG, during follow-up, date in late 1987 by Fusejima et al. [7]. It was generally used as an alternative to coronary angiography and it is the best method for the non-invasive-assessment of coronary graft stenosis. Up to date, DU has shown promising results in pre-OP/post-OP evaluation of IMAs function, regardless of the fact that the proximal portion is predominantly detected rather than distal. Improvements in technology and technique of DU nowadays help us in full-length IMAs detection. Numerous studies show that it is possible to perform ultrasonic flow measurements of IMAs. Measurement of IMAa flow by ultrasound (pre-OP/post-OP) can be performed using linear probes or transthoracic echocardiography (TTE) [8]. Imaging probe is put over the skin and use of commercial gels. The linear probe (suprascapular window) uses a main frequency of 7.5 MHz or more. PW (pulse Doppler) is the main tool in measurement with mandatory adjustment of Doppler steer, angle, and sample volume, as well as other parameters important for optimizing the image, which is in the domain of vascular ultrasound. When recording the IMAs flow by TTE (parasternal window), we use standard TTE probes with main frequency and Doppler frequency of 3.5 MHz or more [9]. The transducer should have high lateral and axial resolutions and depth is often set up to 4 cm.

4.1.2 Recording

The native IMAs vessel or as graft can be visualized either from the supraclavicular fossa or from the parasternal window. In the supraclavicular fossa, IMAs should be searched immediately after division from the subclavian artery, in the same location regardless of whether it was used for bypass or not. The patient is in a supine position in a warm room and the person examining him is behind the patient's head. The hand rests on the bed so that micro-movements can be made in the area of the hand. The movements are from the palm, similar to computer-mouse movements, and the probe is in the left hand. The probe is placed in the left supraclavicular fossa, at an angle of 75–80 degrees. To obtain a proper scan of proximal IMAs we rotate the transducer clockwise and inclining it toward the anterior chest wall to become parallel to the IMA. We use slow micro movement to visualize IMAs at proper angle. The hemodynamics of LIMA is examined around 2.0 cm from the subclavian artery. During vessel search doppler scale should be set to around 20 cm/sec for optimal signal detection. In the parasternal window, the native vessel can be traced along several intercostal spaces. And if the IMA is grafted only in the upper intercostal spaces. Sometimes we cannot find IMAs proximally by this window, except during LAST procedures when we usually harvest the LIMA up to the II intercostal space. Sometimes it is easier to follow native IMAs from the distal end (below the bifurcation) to the prox because there are no ribs there. The best view is in the modified left parasternal window with probe oriented craniocaudally near left sternal border. The patient is in the left lateral decubitus position or supine. Vessel is located within the II–V intercostal space, using the TTE probe. IMA is identified as a tubular structure superficial to the heart and pericardium with color flow directed distally. Hemodynamics is recorded using the Pulsed-Wave Doppler.

Detection of the distal part of the grafted IMAs is also performed through the left parasternal window [9]. The patient is in the left lateral decubitus or supine position. In the long-axis view by using 2D and Color Doppler, the ventricle is first identified, then the space in front of the RVOT and the interventricular sulcus. LIMA is identified first by Doppler and then by PW as a tube with specific biphasic flow toward the apex. It is necessary to set the most favorable angle between the basic Doppler beam and the longitudinal axis of the graft, the SV (sample volume or gate) should be expanded in order to record the flow during the entire cycle or most of the cycle. The possibility of successful detection varies and according to this study, it is as high as 86%. The author states in the explanation that they used a lower-frequency probe (5 MHz).

4.1.3 Measurements

Scicchitano et al. in their research reveals that Doppler Ultrasonography (DU) can be used as a reliable non-invasive technique for follow-up IMA patency, even if it is challenging [8]. Authors show that it is possible to detect severe (>70%) stenosis of the IMA graft by DU during rest by flow curve analysis. In those situations, they found peak diastolic velocity/peak systolic velocity (PDV/PSV) < 0.5 and Diastolic Fraction (DF) < 50% as a reliable marker of stenosis.

Flow in normal coronary arteries predominantly occurs during diastole because myocardial contraction increases vascular resistance. Same is in normal LIMA grafts or moderate stenoses because LIMA grafts allow smooth flow into the recipient artery without turbulence. Also, there is the same diameter of LIMA grafts and native coronary arteries and arterial grafts are controlled by similar autoregulatory mechanisms that allow diameter changes in response to myocardial demands. Opposite to this is in ungrafted internal mammary arteries where flow occurs mainly during systole (as in typical in high resistance peripheral arteries). In severe stenoses LIMA grafts show same flow pattern as in ungrafted LIMA, there is loss of the diastolic flow.

The flow characteristics of IMAs proximally, distally before and after CABG are different, as stated in the study by Goto and et al. [8]. Measurement of the proximal segment was performed through the supraclavicular window with linear probes and the distal segment through the parasternal window with TTE probes. Ultrasound scan of IMAs was possible in 80% of cases for all vessel lengths and 90% for only prox segment [10]. There was a difference in the flow curve of grafted and ungrafted IMAs. In general, the ungrafted IMA has a typical triphasic flow curve like typical muscular circulation, while the grafted one has a low-resistance flow curve like typical parenchymatous circulation. Native IMAs belong to peripheral arteries and have a characteristic highly resistant triphasic (rarely biphasic) flow with a high systolic and low diastolic phase [8]. It is a typical flow of peripheral arteries in which the vascular bed is perfused dominantly during the systole. The first component of the flow curve corresponds to the anterograde flow during systole and is measured by the peak velocity, i.e., peak systolic velocity (PSV). The second component of the flow curve corresponds to the reverse or rejected wave during early diastole and is measured at the maximum speed at the beginning of diastole, i.e., end-diastolic velocity (EDV). Although it is called EDV, it means early diastole. The third component of the flow curve is the later anterograde flow in the end diastole, i.e., Late Diastole Velocity. After IMAs anastomosis with coronary low-resistance circulation, deformation of the flow curve in IMAs occurs. Perfusion is performed dominantly (2/3 of the total blood) in diastole. IMAs then show two peaks in flow: systolic (now smaller) and diastolic (much bigger than before) [8]. The flow amplitude during systole decreases at the expense of an increase in amplitude during diastole. The increase in diastolic flow is the result of blood inflow into the low-resistance coronary vascular bed of the parenchymatous organ - the heart. There are also differences in the flow curve of grafted IMAs proximally and distally. In the proximal part of the graft, the flow is biphasic with a systolic-diastolic component (like the flow in the arterial end of an AV fistula). Other authors such as Federici A. also stated these characteristics in the flow curve along the IMAs graft [11]. At distal end, dominant systolic flow becomes the dominant diastolic flow. In general, this study showed that DU is safe, reliable, and reproducible when it comes to the evaluation of coronary flow through the IMAs graft. Although there are no guidelines that define the reference value for native and grafted IMAs and the distinction between diseased of normal. Several well conducted studies can be used for developing local vascular diagnostic criteria. For example, mentioned authors above quantify flow, resistance index, and diameters of IMAs. In grafted IMAs diameters do not increase significantly (2.21 ± 0.18 vs. 2.27 ± 0.22 mm). There was a significant increase of flow volume in IMAs in the early postoperative period (39.77 ± 21.59 vs. 25.96 ± 13.17 mL/min) and resistance index RI/RI decrease (1.43 ± 0.46 vs. 4.20 ± 1.49). They also compare DU and TTFM: MGF (TTFM) has a moderate correlation with the flow volume on DU. Probably because TTFM was recorded intra-OP and DU post-OP. The same was for PI[10].

What we are interested in when analyzing the flow is the presence of stenoses/ occlusions or competition. The authors described the phenomena and quantified pathologies so that may have a practical place [8]. Evaluation near the anastomosis is the best location to evaluate competitive flow. It is challenging due to the existence of two flows (native and in the graft) and due to myocardial contraction. Evaluation for degree of graft stenosis by DU is possible, but it is unreliable in moderately severe diameter stenoses (50–70%). Because, with these stenoses at rest, the flow velocities do not increase and the basic flow curve value mostly retains the physiological shape. In the case of severe stenoses, there is a deformation of the flow curve. Authors Hata M et al. monitored the correlation of stenoses on angiography and DU and monitored the diameters of IMAs and the characteristics of the curve in stenosis [12]. Doppler waveform along LIMA shows a different pattern from proximal part to the distal one. Trend over time in post-OP period shows LITA diameter increase in the first-month post-CABG (initial diameter 1.71 ± 0.72 vs. diameter after 30 days 1.99 ± 0.31 mm). The diastolic peak velocity and diastolic/systolic velocity ratio (D/S) in the postoperative early phase also increased by 0.26 ± 0.08 m/sec. and 1.54 ± 0.04, respectively. Also, there is a decrease in diastolic peak velocity and D/S ratio of less than 1.0 (D/S ratio > 1.0 was associated with a good angiographic finding).

Also, there is a difference in the flow curve in severe stenoses in the proximal and distal part of the IMA graft. Proximal stenosis (imaging distal to the stenosis) results in a monophasic flow curve with a preserved systolic component (loss of diastolic). This is a typical pathophysiological feature of peripheral artery disease progression. Namely, in the periphery, as the disease progresses, the three-phase curve first disappears and becomes biphasic and then monophasic, and finally the flow stops. On the other hand, the distal stenosis (imaging proximal to the stenosis) retains the biphasic shape due to the elasticity of the IMS, but the diastolic component is reduced. In stenoses of IMAs >75%, there are additional characteristics of the flow curve at PW. First of all, there is an increase in PSV at rest if we are near a stenosis (as a double/triple increase in flow). If, on the other hand, we record an increase in the peak of diastolic velocity (PDV), the risk of graft stenosis is small. There is also the PDV/PSV ratio as a useful marker of the presence of significant stenosis (and it is not dependent on the imaging angle) In case of occlusions, the flow is interrupted (with minimal flow into the occluded graft until it thromboses). Occlusion is present when there is no flow or when we have two sharp curves "to and from" the anastomosis with minimal amplitude. According to the works of Bach et al. a normal IMA graft has an increase in diastolic phase from proximal to distal [13]. The proximal PDV/PSV ratio is 0.6 and the distal ratio is 1.4. The cutoff is >1 as a sign of patent graft. Absence of this increase or reduction of PDV/PSV ratio < 0.5/0.6 is a predictor of severe graft stenosis [14]. These values correlate with angiographic regular findings [12]. The next important parameter of the flow curve of IMAs grafts is Diastolic Fraction (DF). It is the proportion of diastolic flow to the entire flow, i.e., velocity time integral - VTI (i.e., the percentage of the area under the curve that belongs only to diastole). The formula is DF = DVTI/(DVTI + SVTI). Where DVTI is diastolic VTI, DSTI is systolic VTI. The use of DF is more accurate than the absolute value of DVTI, and has less inter and intra-observer variability. A cutoff for hemodynamically significant stenosis (>70%) at rest is DF < 50% [15]. DF significantly positively correlates with invasive measurements [16].

Other authors also described the use of TTE in imaging LIMA grafts [17]. They detect flow in 80% of cases. Flow was biphasic (systolic and diastolic) in normal grafts or if the stenosis is <70%. The biphasic pattern is predominantly diastolic. In stenoses of IMAs >70%, the flow pattern is predominantly systolic. Diastolic fraction (DF) of VTI in normal IMAs and stenosis <70% was 0.81 ± 0.11 and in stenosis >70% it was 0.25 ± 0.06. That is, DF < 0.5 predict severe graft stenosis with a sensitivity and specificity of 100%. Also Ratio PSV/EDV in normal grafts and stenoses <70% was 0.61 ± 0.31 and in stenoses >70% it was 3.21 ± 0.49. This ratio predicted severe stenosis with a sensitivity and specificity of 100 and 90%, respectively.

James J et al. showed that TTE probes can image the IMAs graft in 81% of cases. Such high percentages generally encourage doctors to use non-invasive tools when patients have borderline pathologies or when recurrence of anginal symptoms after CABG is present [18]. Thus, they noticed, like other authors, two flow patterns through the grafts, both of which were biphasic (systolic and diastolic). In a normal graft or moderate (<70%) stenosis, blood flow velocity was maximal during diastole. In patients with native IMA or in severe (>70%) graft stenosis, blood velocity was maximal during systole, and low velocities were recorded during diastole. The diastolic fraction of the velocity time integrals in normal grafts was 0.77 ± 0.07 and 0.27 ± 0.01 in severe stenosis of grafts. A diastolic velocity time integral fraction <0.5 predicted severe stenosis with a sensitivity and specificity of 100%. The ratio of systolic-to-diastolic peak velocities in normal grafts was 0.54 ± 0.26 and 3.45 ± 0.74 in diseased ones. A systolic-to-diastolic peak velocity ratio > 1 predicted severe stenosis with a sensitivity of 100% and specificity of 85%. Authors conclude that TTE allows the identification of the LIMA grafts and measurement of blood flow. Compared with patent grafts or those with moderate lesions, severe stenoses demonstrated different Doppler velocity patterns. Velocity patterns of severely stenosed grafts were similar to those in the ungrafted LIMA control group.

As we can see ultrasound is a totally non-invasive and non-infectious method, unlike coronary angiography. It can also be used to record the functionality of the grafts and the state of the coronary circulation. And simple curve characteristics such as flow rate can be used in the analysis of graft functionality. An example is the study of Hirata et al. which showed blood flow velocity at the anastomotic sites of 83 ± 228 cm/s in stenotic cases and 59 ± 28 cm/s in normal anastomotic cases [17].

4.1.4 Flow reserve

As noted above, flow measurement of IMAs grafts can be performed at rest and during stress testing. This is important because gafted IMAs flow velocities far from stenosis may not be changed in patients with significant stenosis if performed during rest (basal flow). That is why the assessment of the grafted IMAs stenosis is more reliable if we calculate so-called flow reserve. Knowledge from invasive studies transferred to DU can be used in such situations. So, in maximal coronary dilatation, the flow increases much more in normal blood vessels than in stenosed ones (both in ml/min and cm/sec). In this way, moderately severe stenoses can be revealed. Generally, during the stress test, there is an increase in the demand for oxygen, and an auto-regulatory increase in the flow rate, which is a confirmation of the patent graft. Coronary vasodilators such as dipyridamole (which acts on resistance vessels) or nitroglycerin (NTG, which acts on capacitance vessels) can be used for this purpose. With the use of both drugs, the diastolic component of the PDV flow curve increases without an increase in PSV if the findings are normal. Dipyridamole also increases the heart rate and diameter of the LIMA-graft, with increase in vessel capacity. NTG increases PDV in LIMA, without effects on diameter. Some non-pharmacological measures can also affect the flow curve like hyperventilation and Valsalva maneuver (but only in native IMAs). Thus, during hyperventilation, blood velocity increased while during the expiratory effort of the Valsalva maneuver, there is a decrease in mean flow [19]. These changes in flow are also present in TEE measurements of native coronary artery stenoses [20]. Here authors caused a stress test with dipyridamole infusion, and the test showed that there was no increase in flow in any severe stenosis. But, that increase occurs in patent-normal grafts. Dipyridamole baseline PDV and DV ratios were in normal patients on LAD 3.22 ± 0.96 and 3.04 ± 0.88 and in stenosed patients 1.46 ± 0.45 and 1.48 ± 0.49.

Other authors also showed that the DU measurement of IMAs grafts and the stress test represent a simple protocol and have promising results [21]. Constantly present criticisms of minimally invasive direct coronary artery bypass surgery (MIDCAB) in terms of slightly worse graft patency are a good reason to present the results of flow reserve and its connection with graft stenoses. Advances in ultrasound have made it easier to record the flow of IMAs grafts. Monitoring of patency and flow reserve should be part of regular ambulatory monitoring. In this study, flow reserve was measured after adenosine infusion. Patent IMAs grafts had predominantly diastolic flow at rest with PDV 48 ± 20 cm/s, with diastolic TVI 21 ± 10, with PDV/PSV ratio 1.3 ± 0.6, with DF (TVI) of 70% ± 11. Native IMAs (contralateral, high resistance circulation) had a resting flow of PDV/PSV ratio of 0.2 ± 0.1, with a DF (TVI) of 30% ± 10. Occluded IMAs grafts at rest had no flow or a minimal systolic peak was present. After adenosine during the stress test, there is an increase in flow in normal IMAs grafts: aPDV 105 ± 28 cm/s, diastolic TVI 37 ± 19 cm, adenosine/baseline flow ratios of 2.4 ± 0.9 and 2.0 ± 0.7, the diastolic flow velocity reserve was inversely related to baseline diastolic flow.

In the end, we have an interesting statement in the work of Dubey et al. comparing TTE and angiography in measuring severe stenoses of IMAs graft [22]: "It is suggested that angiography may be reserved for cases in which Doppler echocardiography fails to visualize the internal mammary artery or reveals an abnormal flow pattern." Even we may not fully agree with this statement, because the use or exclusion of additional diagnostic tools requires an additional clinical picture. In this paper, the authors compared angiographic data with Doppler echocardiography findings and scintigraphy. They visualized via TTE IMAs in 98% of cases. In 9% there were abnormal angiograms. Thallium scanning in patients with suboptimal angiographic results but non-severe stenosis (4%) showed no evidence of myocardial ischemia in the left anterior descending artery territory.

4.1.5 Limitations

Limitations of the use of DU (pre-OP/post-OP) in the detection of stenosis/occlusion or competitive flow with or without anginal signs are related for several reasons. First one is the staff and second is guidelines/protocols. An expert is needed to monitor the patient pre-OP and post-OP. Even he can miss borderline stenoses if changes in PSV, EDV, and various ratios are not detected at the right spot. Also, error is possible if recordings were not compared with previous or baseline velocities and flow ratios. Due to these limitations, flow monitoring in the grafts should be supplemented by flow monitoring in the venous arm of the coronary circulation (coronary sinus). This volumetric calculation can attenuate hardly detectable marginal stenoses measured at rest and unreachable venous grafts (outside OR). When dealing with guidelines and protocols there are not enough well-conducted studies that compare DU and CT angiography in graft stenosis. However, above mentioned non-invasive measurements can serve as base for local protocol development and for screening of failing grafts or native vessel progression.

4.1.6 Intra-OP

Intraoperatively, the most useful and surgeon-friendly equipment for flow measurement is TTFM. Other vascular Doppler devices can give the same information but use is limited to additional knowledge about vascular ultrasound and flow calculation. TTFM is a device that uses ultrasound media delay for calculation of flow. It does not use Doppler effects (reflection from erythrocytes) for generating flow curves and is widely used outside medicine. The principle of ultrasonic velocity measurement is simple. Probe send signal, through vessel, on opposite side to reflect and return to calculate time delay, giving flow velocity. By using probe with specific diameter device calculate flow in ml/min. The basics of using TTFM are easy to learn [23]. Values that suggest a patent graft are flow >15 c/min, PI <5.0–3.0, and Diastolic Filling 60–80% (for left-sided vessels) and 45–55% (for right-sided vessels). For maximum data extraction multiple measurements are needed. Primarily because early identification of suboptimal grafts and early revision will minimally impact operative quality. Often during OPCAB we perform TTFM after anastomosis with/without proximal snares, with/without stabilizer, and after protamine. In addition to the above, in ONCAB, we measure flow during arrest and on/off pump. But why do we have suboptimal grafts instantly? There are several reasons for instant IMAs graft low/no flow: graft/anastomosis stenosis and competitive flow. The main reason for stenosis is intra-OP errors, which can be repaired by reanastomosing. The main reason for competitive flow is the presence of moderate native vessel stenosis and patent anastomosis per se. Competitive flow reduces the blood flow within the graft and leads to the string phenomenon. Our unpublished experiences show that competition results in occlusion of either a native LAD or LIMA graft within 30 days, and therefore special attention should be paid to it. Clinical importance of those conditions is in protocol consequences. If there is low flow, the surgeon snares the native coronary artery proximally and distally to the anastomosis and record TTFM. If flow increases significantly, it means that competitive flow is present. But, this is often at risk because vessel spasm or plaque mobilization can occur. If flow does not increase then stenosis or low runoff is present. Often surgeon in this situation reanastomose vessel which can improve the blood flow, except if present competitive flow or severe distal vascular bed disease. Differentiation between stenosis and competitive flow using TTFM is difficult because common values that surgeons use are mean flow and PI [24].

Besides them, other data can be extracted from the flow curve for this differentiation. That's: DF, and graft flow FFT (Fast Fourier Transformation) ratio results in F0/H1 and F0/H2 (FO fundamental frequency, H1 first harmonic). The author found that when the cause is competitive flow, there is systolic backflow, and F0/H2 > 14.89. When the cause is anastomotic stenosis, the waveform maintains a bimodal state and F0/H2 is in a normal state - 1.17. So, to avoid unnecessary re-anastomosis it is important to look for additional value during TTFM. In general, as mentioned surgeons look for basic TTFM parameters: mean flow, PI, and DF. Low flow, high PI, and low DF mean graft problem, but, it does not identify cause. For differentiation between competitive flow and stenosis, other data from waveform shape and FFT ratio (especially F0/H2) can be used. They are not available in standard TTFM machines, but new versions will probably overcome that.

4.1.7 Epicardial probes

In addition to flow measurements through the supraclavicular and parasternal windows, DU probe measurements can be used. The authors in this study compared epicardial probe Doppler data with angiography [25]. They revealed that the percentages of systolic and diastolic reverse flow (%sRF, %dRF), as well as PI, were predictors of early postoperative graft failure. They show that mean flow velocity < 12.5 cm/s, %sRF > 9.3%, %dRF > 4.1%, and PI > 4.4 were predictors of early graft failure. Nowadays it is easy to substitute an epicardial probe with a conventional linear ultrasound transducer (under sterile covering). Some manufacturers deliver epicardial probes with TTFM probes. Such an upgrade, in addition to the advantages described below, is very useful when trying to save the LIMA graft at all costs. The most common fear of surgeons is the use of a dissected LIMA versus the fear of discarding a patent LIMA because of discrete hematoma. These two conditions can be differentiated with epicardial probes [26].

Epicardial probes can be used for flow quality control of IMAs or venous bypasses like any other DU probe. But, because of accessibility, we can record the morphology-geometry of the anastomosis with these probes. Rune et al used TTFM and epicardial ultrasound in the analysis of anastomotic geometry. They measured the length of the anastomosis (DA), the diameter of the LIMA (DM), the diameter of the LAD at the toe of the anastomosis (D1) and 5 mm distal to the anastomosis (D2), as well as the ratios between these variables [27]. Flow was analyzed by Doppler and TTFM. They show that it was possible to accurately confirm the patency of anastomoses and that mean ratios of D1/D2, DA/D2, and DM/D2 were 0.89 ± 0.13, 3.01 ± 1.04, and 1.32 ± 0.32, respectively. Those data are useful because they show that anastomosis geometry (orientationally, the length of the anastomosis should be >2 times the diameter of the recipient vessel) correlates with patency.

4.1.8 Graft configuration

Han et al. analyzed different bypass configurations and their effect on coronary flow [28]. Total flows (by TTFM) in IMAs are best when BIMA grafts are used ipsilaterally, i.e., to the corresponding native vessels (LIMA left and RIMA right). If we use BIMA grafts for the left basin, then it does not matter which IMAs feed the LAD (the flow is the same MF, PI, or DF). If we compare the flow in native RIMA with free RIMA, the flow in native RIMA is better. On the other hand, there is no difference in flow and resistance indices (PI, MGF, and DF) through free RIMA (e.g., if it was short or injured) whether it was sutured proximally to the aorta or the LIMA. Olaf et al. analyzed the flow reserve of prox IMAs in composite configurations and showed that it is adequate for second arterial grafts [29].

Shahzad G et al. analyzed the flows in the arms of the composite graft [30]. Generally, the flow reserve of the proximal IMA is sufficient for composite grafts. Namely, in the radial arm of the composite graft, flows of 161 ± 81 mL/min were measured, and in the IMAs arm 137 ± 57 mL/min (together it is 298 ± 101 mL/min). In free flow through both grafts simultaneously, the proximal flow is 226 ± 84 mL/min. It is less by 24 ± 14% compared to the mentioned total flow. The first sum of flow can be considered as maximum and the second sum of flow proximal to the arms as current. After creating the anastomosis, the flow in the radial branch alone was 88 ± 49 mL/min and through the IMAs branch 60 ± 45 mL/min while they had flowed at the same time (measurement before branching, i.e., prox IMAs 140 ± 70 mL/min). Using these numbers, we can determine the surrogate of coronary reserve, i.e., graft flow reserve. Thus, flow reserve (prox IMAs before and after anastomosis with both open branches) is 160%, i.e., 1.6. This flow reserve value is consistent with earlier studies that measured a value of 1.8 during the first week and first month after CABG [31]. In addition to the configuration of the graft, the flow can be affected by subclavian disease or spasm of the IMAs, so it is necessary to carefully handle the graft during harvesting and during the recording of the flow and exceptionally use dilatation instruments for that purpose (probe 1.5 mm).

In addition to assessing the adequate configuration of the grafts in terms of potency for the expected increase in flow, the increased risk for the development of competitive flow should also be taken into account if we use grafts in a composite configuration. Namely, the longer the graft, the lower the perfusion pressure at the end, the longer the delay of the pulse wave, and the greater the risk of developing competition. The consequences of competition are not negligible because competition disturbs the anterograde flow in diastole and the delay of the pulse wave in IMAs promotes retroflow in early systole. The consequences of this oscillating flow around the anastomosis are seen on the endothelium, where NO and prostacyclins are released, causing the string sign, i.e., physiological vasoconstriction of that part of the graft. It usually develops in medium-severe stenoses of native coronary arteries with patent anastomosis and leads to graft or native vessel failure. This phenomenon is even more pronounced with composite grafts because, in addition to the aforementioned anastomoses, they deepen the phase delay of the pulse wave. So that the prevention of competition is related not only to the selection of the target (moderately severe *vs.* severe stenoses) but also to the configuration of the grafts (avoid composite grafts in moderately stenotic coronary arteries, particularly in the RCA territory).

4.1.9 CAD and PAD

Patients with combined coronary artery disease and peripheral artery disease (CAD and PAD), especially severe aortoiliac occlusive pathology, require special caution when selecting grafts [32]. In these conditions, the IMAs represent part of the collateral flow to the lower extremities (e.g., Sy Lerish). So, careful avoidance of IMAs grafts is a wise approach. In all these situations, angiographic visualization of the internal mammary artery is crucial to confirm whether it is involved in collateral circulation or not. The situation is similar for subclavian disease, regardless of whether LIMA-LAD is planned or performed earlier [33]. In order to avoid the development of LAD steal syndrome, it is necessary to systematically examine the IMAs inflow artery.

4.1.10 CAD and PCI

In addition to the intraoperative quality control of the bypass, we have the opportunity to evaluate the flow through the stents. A typical example is RCA stenting in complex and long-term operations. Then when we suspect that the stent has become blocked/bent (during OPCAB manipulations or during valvular surgery). Then, after installing the stabilizer foot, we prepare the native RCA on the most accessible part and measure the flow through TTFM. If everything is normal, the flow is typical diastolic. In our center, the flow measurement of native RCA is performed only by indication.

In addition to the configuration of the grafts and PAD, the measured flow can be affected by the use of CPB. The variations are small but should be kept in mind. In general, the flow is higher and the resistance index is lower with ONCAB (probably on the basis of ischemia and consequent vasodilatation) [34]. Here, the authors quantified OPCAB/ONCAB flow differences. MGF (mean graft flow) was higher in ONCAB versus OPCAB (for all grafts 32 vs 28 mL/min; 30 vs 27 mL/min for arterial grafts and 35 vs 31 mL/min for venous grafts). PI was lower in the ONCAB group (2.1 vs 2.3, for all grafts). Diastolic fraction (DF) was slightly lower in the ONCAB group (65 vs 67.5%). The backflow was also lower in the ONCAB group (0.6 vs 1.3) with trends similar to MGF and PI for venous and arterial grafts. We must not forget that cardiac surgeons sometimes refrain from revising possible stenoses. Because of the above, flow objectification should be daily, especially when we have borderline stenoses.

Other situations that can affect flow in the LIMA graft are therapeutic radiation (in carcinomas). Although we have papers suggesting that the flow is equal, the durability of such grafts is no longer the same as native unirradiated ones which must be kept in mind.

4.2 Venous side of coronary circulation

In order to complete flow evaluation of whole coronary circulation before and after CABG, it is also necessary to quantify changes in coronary sinus flow using noninvasive method (TTE). Of course, we can identify all three coronary arteries and their segments but because of accuracy and reliability, it is easy to measure flow on venous side of coronary circulation—CS blood flow [35]. Another reason is that imaging at the venous side incorporates all new blood from unreachable to DU grafts Post-OP. Currently, there are no TTE-based diagnostic criteria for Ischemic Heart Disease of follow-up. Nor pre or nor post, but there are publications that describe TTE as a screening method for Coronary Artery Disease in isolated populations [36–38]. Quantifications of CS blood flow changes after CABG can be performed using Echocardiography [39–41]. Generally, CS flow increase after CABG for 20% per gram of myocardium per graft [42]. Anny sudden decrease during follow-up period can suggest a new native or bypass flow problem occurrence.

TTE for coronary sinus recording is performed in lateral decubitus position. With B mode, 4 chamber view is used to find CS after dorsal probe angulation. CS can then be found in atrioventricular grove and traced to distal segment. Then probe is rotated until minimal angle of insonation is recorded (about 30 degree). In this position, we have to record VTI with Doppler angle of 60% and in B/M mode diameter of CS under same systemic hemodynamic parameters [43]. After few cardiac cycles, VTI is traced and average value is memorized together with CS diameter and systemic hemodynamic data. For recordings in short axis view the patient is in same position. Distal CS segment is recorded behind mitral valve with minimal probe angulation. Using this view Doppler angle can be even more decreased. Banjanovic B. et al. used following formula for flow calculations [44]: $Q = (VTI \times CSA) \times HR$. Where Q is flow, $(VTI \times CSA)$ is stroke volume, HR is heart rate, CSA = Cross Section Area of CS (πr^2, r = radius if vessel is round), VTI is average velocities calculated automatically after tracing heart cycle velocities. They adopted above formula as $CSA = CSA \times 0{,}39$. Reason for this is ellipsoid shape of cross-section area of CS with a ratio 2:1. As they had recorded a longer cross-section diameter in four-chamber view calculation of cross section area was πab ("a" was half of longer CS diameter, "b" was half of shorter CS diameter that mean "b" was 1/4 of measured diameter).

There are published data about immediate flow changes after CABG recorded using TTE and TEE [2, 42]. Immediate coronary flow increase after triple CABG is up to 50% of native coronary flow. Increase is much higher if there are no microvascular disturbances. Over time, flow increase due to graft and capillary bed vasodilatation. The practical importance of repeated imaging of flow through the CS with TTE is in the trend. Because trend is constant and positive during the early post-OP period. So, any sudden stop in increase or even decrease could lead to suspicion of graft/native vessel failure. That's why Banjanovic et al. performed TTE flow imaging before and two times after CABG (1 and 6 postoperative day [44]. They measure CS diameter, Velocity Time Integral (VTI), and systemic hemodynamic data. Data needed for LV mass calculation were recorded once. The results shown below were obtained at rest due to the careful selection of patients (all patients had at least one severe stenosis of native coronary arteries). They show preoperatively very low CS flow (mean 181 ± 72 ml/min) as others. In published data, we found that normal CS flow is higher (mean 327 ± 125 ml/min). During follow up according to their results there was a constant increase in CS flow from first postoperative day (mean 276 ± 79 ml/min) to last measurement on six postoperative days (mean 355 ± 99 ml/min), in **Figure 1**.

Other published data show even higher immediate postoperative/post-PCI CS flow (mean 451 ± 102 ml/min) [45]. Our understanding of this flow discrepancy is in flow calculation. We take into account ellipsoid shape of terminal CS (2:1) during calculation, so our flow data were less for 0,39 times. Also using angle of 60 degrees during the Doppler VTI calculation brings us with error of 10%. CS flow discrepancy could be because of recording position wary in terminal CS segment from patient to patient. But this was probably nullified by repeated measurements, as it will be during future follow-up in outpatient departments. According to the literature, net flow through three grafts after CABG is about 110–130 ml/min. As net native coronary artery flow is about 250 ml/min during rest, volume of new blood in coronary artery bed after CABG is 50% of net native flow during rest [2, 46]. For even more individualization of results, they performed CS flow calculation over LV mass. They found preoperatively low CS flow per gram of LV (mean 0,68 ± 0,30 ml/gram/min). Which corresponds to invasive

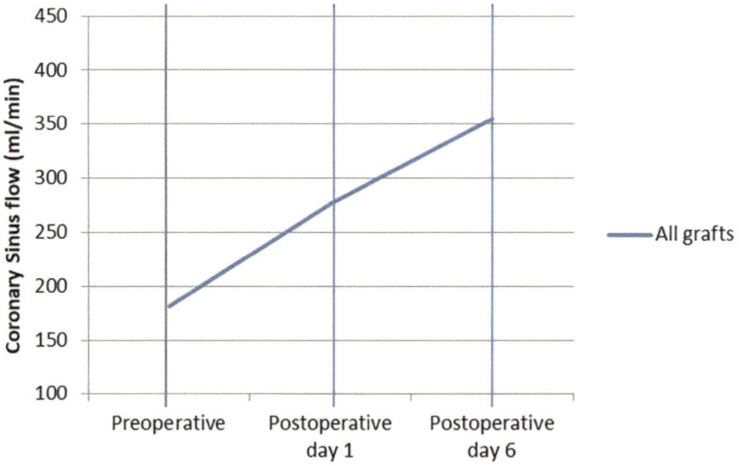

Figure 1.
Flow through CS during repeated measurements (ml/min), after CABG.

measurements. And there was also CS flow increase over time per gram of LV, from day 1 mean flow 1,13 ± 0,35 ml/gram/min to day 6 mean flow 1,30 ± 0,46 ml/gram/min. All data above support correct indication for CABG because coronary vessel bed was empty and constantly filled with new blood in following 6 days. Other variables recorded were: CS diameter was preoperatively mean 7,5 ± 1,1 mm, first postoperative day mean 8,2 ± 1,4 mm, and 6 postoperative days 9,3 ± 1,3 mm. As flow is proportional to the forth square of diameter, those changes can have huge impact on flow calculations. In this paper, calculation error was decreased three times by fact that we record elliptic segment of CS. Heart rate also has a direct positive impact in flow calculations. In our results, heart rate increase from mean 68 (±8,9) preoperatively to 87 (±11) first and same at the sixth postoperative day. As heart rate was constant postoperatively, the impact on error in flow calculation was decreased in **Table 1**.

	Preoperative	1 postoperative day	6 postoperative day
Flow $_{(VTI\ syst\ +\ diast)}$ ml/min	181 (±72)	276 (±79)	355 (±99)
Flow $_{(VTI\ syst\ +\ diast)}$ ml/min/per I graft	120 (±10)	240 (±69)	232 (±55)
Flow $_{(VTI\ syst\ +\ diast)}$ ml/min/per II graft	175 (±65)	281 (±94)	378 (±89)
Flow $_{(VTI\ syst\ +\ diast)}$ ml/min/per III graft	186 (±78)	269 (±52)	352 (±100)
Flow $_{(VTI\ syst\ +\ diast)}$ ml/min/per IV graft	234 (±43)	379 (±165)	448 (±8)
Flow $_{(VTI\ syst\ +\ diast)}$ ml/gram LV	0,68 (±0,30)	1,13 (±0,35)	1,30 (±0,46)
CS VTI $_{(syst\ +\ diast)}$	12,0 cm (±3,4)	11,9 cm (±3,9)	12,2 cm (±3,3)
CS VTI $_{(max)}$	35 cm (±7,7)	41 cm (±14,5)	34 cm (±5,9)
CS diameter	7,5 mm (±1,1)	8,2 mm (±1,4)	9,3 mm (±1,3)
Heart rate	68 (±8,9)	87 (±11)	87 (±11)

CS-Coronary Sinus LV-left ventricle, RV-right ventricle.

Table 1.
Flow through CS during repeated measurements after CABG.

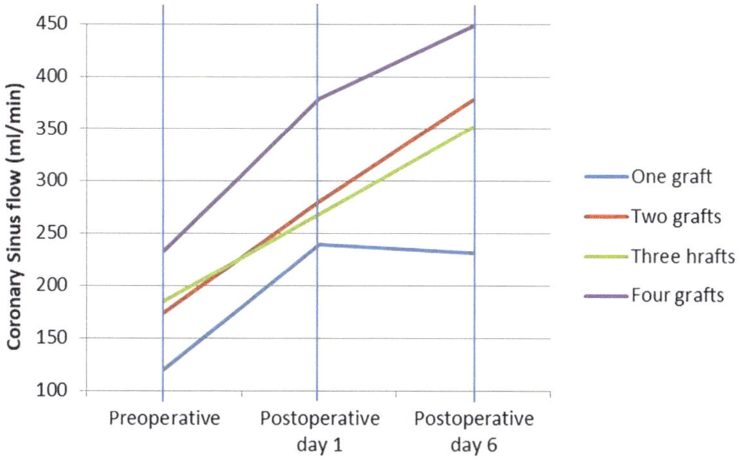

Figure 2.
CS flow comparison during repeated measurements, effect of graft number.

Authors show that it is possible to detect effect of graft number on CS flow. That there is evidence of maximal amount of new blood in the coronary bed after four bypasses and that same amount of new blood was whatever the patient gets three or two grafts, in **Figure 2**. Meaning that the increase in flow by graft number is linear at the beginning and after that is stepwise.

5. Conclusion

Functional evaluation of each graft is crucial during the follow-up of patients who underwent CABG intervention. The gold standard investigation for the assessment of conduit stenosis remains CA, but this is an invasive technique with many risks. Different non-invasive methods had been recently developed for coronary graft evaluation.

DU seems to be the best non-invasive tool to assess graft patency and coronary sinus flow. In the early post-OP after CABG there is a constant increase in coronary flow. The increase is significant overall after classifying per gram of LV and graft number. That's why measurements via DU should cover IMAs grafts, coronary sinus and include intra-OP TTFM measurements of all other grafts (GSV/SSV or radial artery). This means that intra-OP (TTFM) graft flow measurements must be available to outpatient departments.

What data should be recorded for stenosis or competition evaluation? For practical use depending on used equipment that's are as show below. For DU—IMA native/grafts diameter: PSV, EDC, PSV/EDV, EDV/PSV, DF, ml/min, PI/RI, VTIsistolic, VTI diastolic, heart rate. For DU—coronary sinus: VTI, diameter, ml/min. For TTFM—all grafts: ml/min, PI/RI diastolic filling, retro flow pik. For epicardial probe: all grafts: same as for DU and %sRF, % dRF, D1-anastomotic length, D0-vessel diameter, ratio D1/D0.

DU has good reproducibility, ease of use, and significant correlation with angiographic results which make DU the best technique to be adopted in clinical ambulatory practice in order to follow-up with patients who underwent CABG. Thus, the periodicity of flow measurement should be regularly increased from weeks to every 6 months.
If during follow-up period flow decrease or a flow curve deform that is indication of the disease progression. In the situation we should offer a re-evaluation to all patients depending on clinical picture (e.g. ERGO, scintigraphy or coronary re-angiography, etc.).

Author details

Bedrudin Banjanović[1*], Edin Kabil[1], Nedžad Kadrić[2], Emir Mujanović[2], Mirza Dilić[3], Mehmed Kulić[4], Samed Djedović[2], Amel Hadžimegmedagić[1], Muhamed Djedović[1], Zina Lazović[1], Sevleta Avdić[2], Tarik Selimović[1], Lejla Divović[1] and Nada Malešić[1]

1 Clinic for Cardiovascular Surgery, University Clinical Center Sarajevo, Bosnia and Herzegovina

2 Medical Institute Bayer, Tuzla, Bosnia and Herzegovina

3 Clinic for Heart Disease, Blood Vessels and Rheumatism, University Clinical Center Sarajevo, Bosnia and Herzegovina

4 Cardioteam Clinic, Sarajevo, Bosnia and Herzegovina

*Address all correspondence to: bedrudinx10@gmail.com

References

[1] Lokeswara R. A narrative review of redo coronary artery bypass grafting. AME Medical Journal. 2021;**6**:20

[2] Hajaghaei M, Maleki M, Salehi HR, Ojaghi Z, Noohi F. Coronary flow reserve measurement in the coronary sinus in pre and post CABG status. Iranian Cardiovascular Research Journal. 2007;**1**:2

[3] Tamilselvi R, Henry S. Coronary blood flow. Continuing Education in Anaesthesia. Critical Care and Pain. 2005;**5.2**:61-64

[4] Partha G. A Clinical Review of Myocardial Blood Flow and Coronary Flow Reserve with Dynamic Myocardial Perfusion PET/CT. 2010. Available from: www.siemens.com/mi

[5] Dimitrow PP, Galderisi M, Rigo F. The non-invasive documentation of coronary microcirculation impairment: Role of transthoracic echocardiography. Cardiovascular Ultrasound. 2005;**3**:18

[6] Mady EN, Whitelaw S, Gornik HL. Expected diameter and velocity parameters for internal mammary artery mapping procedures. Journal for Vascular Ultrasound. 2009;**33**(3):133-137

[7] Fusejima K. Noninvasive measurement of coronary artery blood flow using combined two-dimensional and Doppler echocardiography. Journal of the American College of Cardiology. 1987;**10**(5):1024-1031

[8] Scicchitano P, De Palo M, Parisi G, Gioia MI, Ciccone MM. Doppler ultrasound selection and follow-up of the internal mammary artery as coronary graft. Biomedicine. 2023;**11**(1):66

[9] El-Masry MM, Salama MM, Darwish AZ, Abd E-AO. Assessment of left internal mammary artery graft patency by transthoracic Doppler echocardiography. Clinical Cardiology. 2002;**25**(11):511-516

[10] Junxue G, Zhou Z, Jiaan Z, Hui T, Yuejie L. The role of color Doppler ultrasonography in the perioperative period of coronary artery bypass grafting: Comparison with transit-time flow measurement. Cardiology. 2021;**146**(5):583-590

[11] Federici A, Ciccone M, di Noia D, Selvaggi G, Antonelli G, Rizzon P. Valutazione incruenta del flusso coronarico mediante ultrasonografia Doppler dell'arteria mammaria interna anastomizzata coronaria sinistra durante sforzo isometrico [the noninvasive assessment of coronary flow during isometric exercise by Doppler ultrasonography of the internal mammary artery anastomosed to the left coronary]. Cardiologia. 1993;**38**(9):555-559

[12] Hata M, Raman JS, Shiono M, Sezai A, Negishi N, Sezai Y, et al. What can Doppler wave forms of the left internal thoracic artery teach us? the efficacy of apical transthoracic approach of Doppler echocardiography. Annals of Thoracic and Cardiovascular Surgery. 2002;**8**(2):92-96

[13] Bach RG, Kern MJ, Donohue TJ, Aguirre FV, Caracciolo EA. Comparison of phasic blood flow velocity characteristics of arterial and venous coronary artery bypass conduits. Circulation. 1993;**88**(5 Pt 2):II133-II140

[14] Mizukami N, Kisanuki A, Hamasaki S, Takasaki K, Yuasa T, Kuwahara E, et al. Different flow patterns between left and right

internal thoracic artery grafts influence the evaluation of severe graft stenosis by transthoracic Doppler echocardiography. Journal of the American Society of Echocardiography. 2011;**24**(7):768-774

[15] Leitão MC, Lobo Filho JG, Freire TM, Montenegro ML, Jamacuru FV, Carvalho ER, et al. Doppler echocardiographic criteria in patency assessment of composite grafts from left internal thoracic artery. Revista Brasileira de Cirurgia Cardiovascular. 2013;**28**(2):167-175

[16] Takagi T, Yoshikawa J, Yoshida K, Akasaka T, Maeda K. Noninvasive measurement of left internal mammary artery bypass graft flow by duplex Doppler echocardiography from the supraclavicular fossa. Journal of the American Society of Echocardiography. 1993;**6**(4):374-381

[17] Hirata N, Asaoka N, Amemiya A, Hatsuoka S, Ueno T, Kosakai Y. Noninvasive evaluation of internal thoracic artery and left anterior descending coronary artery anastomotic sites using transthoracic Doppler echocardiography: Comparison with coronary arteriography. The Journal of Thoracic and Cardiovascular Surgery. 2003;**126**(4):1080-1086

[18] Crowley JJ, Shapiro LM. Noninvasive assessment of left internal mammary artery graft patency using transthoracic echocardiography. Circulation. 1995;**92**:25-30

[19] Ciccone M, Federici A, di Michele L, Marchese A, Chiddo A, Rizzon P. Doppler continuous-wave analysis of grafted mammary artery as a non-invasive technique for static and dynamic assessment of coronary flow in man. European Journal of Applied Physiology and Occupational Physiology. 1990;**61**(5-6):338-343

[20] Iliceto S, Marangelli V, Memmola C, Rizzon P. Transesophageal Doppler echocardiography evaluation of coronary blood flow velocity in baseline conditions and during dipyridamole-induced coronary vasodilation. Circulation. 1991;**83**(1):61-69

[21] Katz WE, Zenati M, Mandarino WA, Cohen HA, Gorcsan J 3rd. Assessment of left internal mammary artery graft patency and flow reserve after minimally invasive direct coronary artery bypass. The American Journal of Cardiology. 1999;**84**(7):795-801

[22] Dubey B, Bhan A, Choudhary SK, et al. Assessment of internal mammary artery graft patency: Angiography or Doppler? Asian Cardiovascular and Thoracic Annals. 2000;**8**(4):325-329

[23] Kieser TM, Taggart DP. The use of intraoperative graft assessment in guiding graft revision. The Annals of Cardiothoracic Surgery. 2018;**7**(5):652-662

[24] Mao B, Feng Y, Duan M, Dong Y, Li G, Li B, et al. A novel method to determine the cause of left internal mammary artery instant non-patency based on transit time flow measurement. Frontiers in Physiology. 2022;**13**:901280

[25] Shinya T et al. Real-time graft flow assessment using epigraftic ultrasonography during coronary artery bypass grafting. European Journal of Cardio-Thoracic Surgery. 2014;**46**(4):706-712

[26] Banjanović B, Bergsland J, Mujanović E, Kabil E. Importance of full-length scan of arterial grafts in coronary artery bypass grafting. Innovations. 2015;**10**(5):352-353

[27] Rune H, Nicola V, Ole T, Arve T, Hans T, Stein O. Intraoperative color

Doppler ultrasound assessment of LIMA-to-LAD anastomoses in off-pump coronary artery bypass grafting. The Annals of Thoracic Surgery. 2002;**74**(4):1390-1394

[28] Han Z, Zhang G, Chen S, et al. Application of bilateral internal mammary artery with different configurations in coronary artery bypass grafting. Journal of Cardiothoracic Surgery. 2021;**16**:2

[29] Olaf W, Benno H, Torsten M, Jochem K, Dietmar T, Qi H, et al. T grafts with the right internal thoracic artery to left internal thoracic artery versus the left internal thoracic artery and radial artery: Flow dynamics in the internal thoracic artery main stem. The Journal of Thoracic and Cardiovascular Surgery. 1999;**118**(5):841-848

[30] Raja SG. Total arterial coronary grafting: Outcomes, concerns and controversies. Vessel Plus. 2019;**3**:23

[31] Wendler O, Hennen B, Markwirth T, König J, Tscholl D, Huang Q, et al. T grafts with the right internal thoracic artery to left internal thoracic artery versus the left internal thoracic artery and radial artery: Flow dynamics in the internal thoracic artery main stem. The Journal of Thoracic and Cardiovascular Surgery. 1999;**118**(5):841-848

[32] Ben-Dor I, Waksman R, Satler LF, Bernardo N, Torguson R, Li Y, et al. A further word of caution before using the internal mammary artery for coronary revascularization in patients with severe peripheral vascular disease! Catheterization and Cardiovascular Interventions. 2010;**75**(2):195-201

[33] Večeřa J et al. Non-invasive diagnosis of coronary-subclavian steal: role of the Doppler ultrasound. European Journal of Echocardiography. 2010;**11**(9):E34

[34] Dror B, Carlo M, Miriam M, Andrea A, Daniel J, Gabriele G, et al. Graft flow evaluation with intraoperative transit-time flow measurement in off-pump versus on-pump coronary artery bypass grafting. JTCVS Techniques. 2022;**15**:95-106

[35] Krzanowski M, Bodzon W, Dimitrow PP. Imaging of all three coronary arteries by transthoracic echocardiography: An illustrated guide. Cardiovascular Ultrasound 2003;1:16

[36] Vrublevsky AV. Reduced coronary flow reserve in the coronary sinus is a predictor of hemodynamically significant stenoses of the left coronary artery territory. European Journal of Echocardiography. 2004;**5**(4):294-303

[37] Zheng X-Z. Coronary sinus flow is reduced and recovered with time in viral myocarditis mimicking acute coronary syndrome. Journal of Ultrasound in Medicine. 2016;**35**:63-69

[38] Zheng X-Z, Yang B, Jing W. Sex-specific assessment of reduced coronary sinus flow in non-hypertensive patients with coronary artery disease at rest. Libyan Journal of Medicine. 2013;**8**(1):21553

[39] Watanabe N. Noninvasive assessment of coronary blood flow by transthoracic Doppler echocardiography: Basic to practical use in the emergency room. Journal of Echocardiography. 2017;**15**:49

[40] Patrick M, Christophe T. Non-invasive assessment of coronary flow and coronary flow reserve by transthoracic Doppler echocardiography: A magic tool for the real world. European Journal of Echocardiography. 2008;**9**:449-457

[41] Sharif D. Detection of severe left anterior descending coronary artery stenosis by transthoracic evaluation of

resting coronary flow velocitydynamics. Heart International. 2010;**5**(2):e10

[42] Tuomas OK, Markku S, Juha WK, et al. Coronary artery diameter can be assessed reliably with transthoracic echocardiography. American Journal of Physiology. Heart and Circulatory Physiology. 2004;**286**:H1515-H1520

[43] Ghassan SK. Functional hierarchy of coronary circulation: Direct evidence of a structure-function relation. American Journal of Physiology. Heart and Circulatory Physiology. 2005;**289**:H2559-H2565

[44] Banjanovic B, Karabic IH, Straus S, Granov N, Kabil E, Jakirlic M, et al. Non invasive detection of coronary sinus flow changes over time after CABG. Acta Informatica Medica. 2022;**30**(3):220-224

[45] Xiaozhi Z, Ping J, Hongwei M, Jianquan H. Reduced anterograde flow in the coronary sinus is a predictor od coronary artery stenosis in hypertensive patients. Journal of Ultrasound in Medicine. 2012;**31**(1):7-14

[46] Scanlon PJ, Faxon DP, Audet AM, et al. ACC/AHA guidelines for coronary angiography: Executive summary and recommendations. Circulation. 1999;**99**:2345-2357

Chapter 4

Perspective Chapter: Right Ventricular Free Wall – The Forgotten Territory for Revascularization

Haytham Elgharably, Serge C. Harb, Amgad Mentias, Khaled Ziada and Faisal G. Bakaeen

Abstract

Revascularization of the right ventricle free wall is not routinely addressed during coronary bypass surgery, yet the clinical impact is not well studied. Addressing right ventricular free wall ischemia is feasible via bypassing branches of the right coronary artery. In this article, we aim to examine the hypothesis that ignoring the right ventricular free wall ischemia during coronary artery bypass surgery could have an early, and possibly late, clinical impact, such as right ventricular dysfunction and functional tricuspid regurgitation, in patients with extended right coronary artery disease without adequate collateralization from the left coronary system. We present the current available evidence that is relevant to that hypothesis.

Keywords: right ventricle, ischemia, right coronary artery, marginal branches, revascularization

1. Introduction

One of the motivations for our hypothesis is a recent case of acute right ventricular (RV) dysfunction after coronary artery bypass grafting (CABG) that resolved after bypassing the right coronary artery (RCA) in the atrio-ventricular groove [1]. The patient was an 82-year-old woman who presented with coronary artery disease, including extended RCA disease, a tight mid-lesion, and another long, tight lesion in the distal part of the artery. There was one large, acute marginal branch in between the two lesions supplying the RV-free wall. There were no robust collaterals between the left and right coronary circulations. She underwent revascularization of the left coronary system lesions as well as the posterior descending artery (PDA). However, upon separation from the cardiopulmonary bypass, she developed new acute RV dysfunction that did not resolve with prolonged reperfusion on the pump and required an increased dosage of inotropes and pressors to support the hemodynamics. After excluding all other possible etiologies, we decided to add a bypass to the RCA in the atrio-ventricular groove between the mid and distal lesions, with the aim to provide blood flow to the RV-free wall through a large acute marginal branch. Only after adding the bypass to the mid-RCA, the RV dysfunction resolve, and the patient required minimal pharmacological support. The patient made a complete recovery with normal RV function at 3 months of follow-up [1].

In addition to this case, it's our clinical observation that similar patients with extended RCA disease and no adequate collateral from the left coronary system, would require higher blood pressure to maintain RV-free wall perfusion, which can be achieved with pharmacological support or an intra-aortic balloon pump. Although this approach may not have a clinical impact in some patients, it could pose a complication risk in older patients with peripheral arterial or kidney disease. In a large cohort study from the Netherlands that included 1109 patients who underwent cardiac surgery, postoperative RV dysfunction (RV ejection fraction <20%) was associated with complicated intensive care unit courses, including prolonged stay, longer duration of mechanical ventilation, higher dosage of inotropes, and higher rates of acute kidney dysfunction [2]. In a similar study from France, out of 3826 patients who underwent cardiac surgery between 2016 and 2019, 3% developed postoperative RV failure with worse outcomes [3]. In addition to the early impact after surgery, not addressing RV-free wall ischemia in patients undergoing CABG could have a late effect. Several studies have reported the persistence of RV dysfunction later after CABG during follow-up [4–7]. Moreover, other studies have shown that RV-free wall revascularization prevented postoperative RV dysfunction and peri-operative ischemic complications [8–10]. In this article, we aim to examine the available relevant evidence to address the question of how important RV-free wall revascularization during CABG is.

2. Coronary revascularization

CABG has been the standard surgical intervention for coronary artery disease for over 50 years [11, 12]. The practice of CABG has been dedicated primarily to address coronary artery pathology with respect to the left ventricular territories (anterior, lateral, and inferior walls), while less commonly to address RV ischemia. This is supported by the current guidelines that focus on the indications for revascularization and different approaches to address left main or multi-vessels disease, yet there are no specific recommendations regarding RV ischemic disease [13, 14]. The evolution in the practice of CABG has been directed toward the utilization of cardiopulmonary bypass versus off-pump, minimally invasive approaches, conduit selection, and harvesting [11, 12, 15]. Completeness of revascularization has been an important focus of CABG, as the outcomes of incomplete revascularization have been shown to be inferior to complete revascularization [13, 16, 17]. However, there is no established definition of complete revascularization, and it continues to be variable across different studies or guideline recommendations. In general, complete revascularization is reported as bypassing coronary vessels with >50% stenosis in the major territories and vessel diameter > 1.5 mm [13, 16, 17]. However, revascularization of the RV-free wall in cases with extended RCA disease has not been specifically considered in the definitions of complete revascularization. Thus, addressing RCA disease commonly includes bypassing the PDA or posterolateral ventricular (PLV) branch and less commonly includes bypassing acute marginal branches or main RCA for extended disease, which could include multi-stenotic lesions or complete occlusion.

3. The forgotten territory in CABG: the RV-free wall

Anatomically, the RV is composed of three components: (1) inflow through tricuspid valve and sub-valvular apparatus (2), trabecular apex, and (3) outflow or infundibulum [18–20]. In cross-section, the RV-free wall, which is part of the ventricular wall not in contact with the interventricular septum, appears as a crescent over the left ventricle (LV) and is composed of anterior, lateral, and inferior walls [19, 20]. The RCA provides the primary blood supply to the RV wall through marginal branches to the lateral wall, and PDA to the inferior wall and posterior one-third of the interventricular septum. The RV anterior wall is supplied by the left anterior descending artery while the infundibulum is supplied by the conal artery [18, 19]. Bowers et al. studied the flow in RCA branches in 125 patients presenting with inferior myocardial infarction secondary to RCA disease [21]. They reported that RCA branch perfusion was critical for RV global performance as proximal lesions resulted in significant RV dysfunction. Spontaneous reperfusion or presence in collaterals maintained the flow in the RV branches which resulted in the preservation of RV function [21]. On echocardiographic imaging of the RV, one of the standard views used for assessment of the RV function is the apical four chambers view, in which the RV-free wall is the anatomical lateral wall supplied by RCA marginal branches [19, 20]. The ejection performance of the RV is based on three mechanisms: inward movement of the free wall (bellows effect), longitudinal shortening that brings tricuspid annulus toward the apex, and stretching of the free wall over the septum secondary to left ventricular contraction [18]. The contribution of each mechanism to RV pump function may vary in different pathological conditions [22]. Recent studies are suggesting for equal contribution of longitudinal and radial movements to global RV performance [23].

4. RV-free wall revascularization

In a pioneer work by Dr. Vineberg in 1968, he reported implanting the right internal mammary artery in the RV myocardium to treat RCA disease in 15 patients [24]. The authors reported no operative mortality or late death during 7 to 22 months of follow-up. In 1988, Drs. Rich, Akins, and Daggett from Massachusetts General Hospital wrote an editorial discussing the possible etiologies for RV dysfunction after cardiopulmonary bypass, ignoring RV revascularization as a possible important etiology [25]. The authors followed a complete RV revascularization approach that includes bypassing disease RCA branches and reported no early or late RV failure in two different cohorts regardless of the technique of the myocardial protection. However, this approach was not widely adopted among cardiac surgeons in the current practice. This could be related to the development of collaterals between the right and left coronary arteries in patients with chronic occlusive disease of the RCA which reduces the incidence of significant RV dysfunction after CABG. Cho et al. reported a case of ischemic tricuspid regurgitation (TR) that improved after revascularization of the left anterior descending artery that provided collateral blood supply to the ischemic region of the RV-free wall [26]. Conversely, if ischemic TR developed in the absence of collaterals between right and left coronary arteries, revascularization of RCA has been shown to improve the TR [27].

Multiple surgical groups from Turkey have adopted the concept of RV-free wall revascularization and studied the impact on clinical outcomes [8–10]. In a prospective randomized study, Güney and Eren compared complete RV revascularization with multiple bypasses to RCA branches (n = 32 patients) to a single conventional bypass to RCA (n = 32 patients) [9]. The authors have demonstrated that complete RV revascularization had a protective effect against peri-operative ischemic events in the RCA territory in patients with ejection fraction <50%. In another study of 35 patients with diffuse atherosclerotic disease of the RCA who underwent CABG; RV diastolic function by echocardiography improved in 20 patients with sequential bypass to RCA compared to 15 patients with single bypass to RCA [10]. In another comparative analysis conducted by Sahin et al., 100 patients with multi-segments disease of the RCA underwent off-pump CABG, in which 50 patients had single bypass to distal RCA and 50 patients had additional bypass to marginal branch of RCA [8]. Patients who had additional bypass to the RV branch experienced faster recovery of RV function, less inotropic support, and shorter hospitalization than the group with single distal RCA bypass.

5. RV dysfunction after CABG

Several properties may render RV less susceptible to ischemia compared to LV, including smaller muscle mass and milder workload resulting in less oxygen requirements [26, 28]. More importantly, in patients with chronic coronary artery disease, rich collaterals develop between the left and right coronary systems and disease of the left coronary system may contribute to RV infarction [26]. This could explain in part the reason that early RV dysfunction is not common after CABG and did not receive increased attention over the evolution of CABG techniques. It could occur in cases with extended RCA disease (complete occlusion, diffuse disease, multi-segment stenosis) without adequate collaterals from the left coronary system while the patient underwent only conventional bypass of distal RCA or PDA [1]. On the other hand, little data is available about the fate of RV recovery after CABG in cases with extended RCA disease.

Roshanali et al. studied RV function after CABG in 240 patients using an echocardiographic assessment of the RV-free wall [4]. In their cohort, 60% had proximal RCA stenosis and 40% had distal RCA stenosis, but they did not elaborate on the details of the proximal RCA disease if it was complete occlusion or multi-segment disease. They reported depressed RV function on echocardiographic assessment up to 1 year after CABG, regardless of the status of RCA bypass which included only bypass to PDA or PLV branch [4]. In a two-part study, Yadav et al. have shown selective RV dysfunction following CABG compared to LV function using Myocardial tissue Doppler velocities to assess ventricular function [5]. The first part was a prospective study of 20 patients undergoing CABG with preoperative and 3-month postoperative echocardiograms. The second part was a retrospective analysis of 101 patients with established heart failure diagnosis, out of which 40 patients had previous CABG. In both parts of the study, the echocardiographic assessment of ventricular function showed a lower RV: left ventricular ratio. Interestingly, they reported the same observation even when CABG patients compared to patients with ischemic pathology of heart failure [5]. In another recent prospective study, Chinikar et al. studied RV function in 61 patients before and after CABG using echocardiographic assessment as well as functional capacity [6]. They found a high frequency of RV dysfunction at 1 week and 6 months after CABG as well as impaired exercise capacity. In that study cohort, 88.5% had RCA disease, 23% had RV branch disease, and 73% received RCA graft but the report did not indicate which part of the RCA or which branch was bypassed or the status of the bypass grafts [6].

6. Ischemic tricuspid regurgitation

Our group has studied the concept of "ischemic TR" in a cohort of ischemic MR patients (n = 568) undergoing mitral valve surgery and CABG +/– tricuspid valve repair [29]. The characteristics of TR in this cohort of patients mimic the characteristics of ischemic MR with dilated annulus, tethered leaflets, and RV dysfunction. However, in longitudinal analysis of left- versus right-sided heart remodeling in the same cohort of patients, we observed an important difference; the LV underwent reverse remodeling with regression in size and recovery of ejection fraction with stable MR over time after surgery [7]. Conversely, the RV continued to dilate with worsening RV function and increased recurrence of TR over time up to 5 years after surgery, even in patients who underwent TV repair. In this cohort, 83% of patients had >50% stenosis of the RCA system, 48% had total occlusion, and 73% of patients underwent bypass of RCA lesion [29]. However, there was no available granular data regarding the extent of the RCA disease (proximal, distal, multi-segment, presence of collaterals with left system) nor the location of the bypass graft to the RCA. Given the common practice of CABG among the surgeons, it is expected that most of the bypass graft to RCA in this cohort was to distal RCA branches such as PDA or PLV branches, and to a lesser extent to include bypass to acute marginal branches. In that sense, even though it is speculation, ignoring the RV-free wall revascularization in some of these patients could have contributed to progressive RV remodeling secondary to chronic ischemia. This could provide an explanation for the difference in recovery between the left ventricle and right ventricle after addressing the mitral valve disease and the coronary artery disease that commonly is dedicated to address the ischemia of the LV territories and to a lesser extent the RV-free wall ischemia.

Onorati et al. had similar findings in a smaller cohort of patients (n = 64) who underwent CABG and mitral valve repair for ischemic MR during a shorter follow-up period of 6 months after surgery [30]. They suggested that patients who needed tricuspid repair had already advanced stage of RV cardiomyopathy as the reason for the failure of RV reverse remodeling compared to the LV. Another group has shown progression of functional TR in patients with dilated cardiomyopathy (the majority were ischemic) after repair of functional MR +/– CABG [31, 32]. In a recent study that included data from two prospective randomized ischemic MR trials, progression of non-severe TR was found to be infrequent while patients with > moderate TR at 2-year follow-up had significant clinical events [33]. This study included 492 patients, with 59% undergoing CABG, while 41% did not require CABG at the time of mitral valve surgery, and 66% of patients having echocardiographic data analysis at a 2-year follow-up. Only 15% of patients required bypass to the RCA [33]. However, these former reports did not indicate details about the extent of the RCA disease or the location and patency of the bypass to the RCA system.

In another longitudinal analysis study, but after percutaneous coronary intervention (PCI), Koren et al. followed the evolution of functional TR in 134 patients presented with ischemic MR after myocardial infarction for a median follow-up of 5 years [34]. They excluded all other etiologies of TR such as primary tricuspid valve pathology, pulmonary hypertension, or RV leads. At the time of the index event of myocardial infarction, 30% of patients developed functional TR, and failed revascularization was an independent predictor for the development and severity of functional TR. In their analysis, there was no association between the development of functional TR and infarct-related arteries or the existence of multi-vessel coronary artery disease. In their cohort, 36% had RCA disease but no available data about the extent of the disease or status of acute marginal branches or collaterals from the left coronary system. During follow-up, functional TR continues to progress in 97.5% of the patients with newly developed functional TR after the index event. The functional TR progression rate was highest in patients with moderate to severe RV dysfunction, > moderate MR, pulmonary hypertension, and LV dysfunction [34].

7. Reoperation for isolated tricuspid regurgitation

One critical question we aim to highlight in this article is: could ignoring the RV-free wall revascularization at the time of CABG have a late clinical impacts, such as RV dysfunction and functional TR in patients with extended RCA disease? Patients

Study	Trans-catheter Intervention	History of CAD, PCI, CABG
Besler et al. [37] (n = 117)	MitraClip	Previous PCI 32% Previous CABG 16%
Fam et al. [38] (n = 28)	PASCAL	CAD 46% PreviousPCI 18% Previous CABG 18%
Kodali et al. [39] (n = 34)	PASCAL	CAD 32% Previous PCI 21% Previous CABG 29%
Nickenig et al. [40] (n = 30)	Cardioband	CAD 37% Previous PCI 20% Previous CABG 23%
Davidson et al. [41] (n = 30)	Cardioband	CAD 13% Previous PCI 27% Previous CABG 3%
Nickenig et al. [42] (n = 61)	Cardioband	CAD 12% Previous PCI 23% Previous CABG 8%
Hahn et al. [43] (n = 15)	Trialign	Previous PCI 7% Previous CABG 27%
Hahn et al. [44] (n = 30)	Navigate	Previous MI 27% Previous PCI 17% Previous CABG 33%
Fam et al. [45] (n = 25)	Evoque	CAD 28% Previous PCI 8% Previous CABG 20%

Table 1.
Prevalence of coronary artery disease in patients undergoing transcatheter intervention for tricuspid regurgitation.

presenting for surgery for isolated tricuspid regurgitation, especially in the setting of reoperation after previous CABG, are often considered high-risk and likely will not be offered another surgery. This could be related to the high mortality rates reported among different groups [35]. These patients commonly present with clinical right heart failure manifestations secondary to RV dysfunction, including liver congestion, renal dysfunction, thrombocytopenia, and volume overload, which adds to the risk of the operation in addition to the technical aspects of re-operation after CABG with patent grafts. In that sense, there might be a group of patients developing right heart failure late after a CABG procedure who will not be referred to the surgeons by the cardiologists, knowing they are high-risk patients. In the current era of evolving trans-catheter therapies, a number of high-risk surgical patients could be referred to tricuspid valve catheter therapies [36]. History of coronary artery disease, PCI, and/or CABG with RV dysfunction can be observed in the reports of trans-catheter tricuspid valve intervention along with common etiologies of functional TR such as pulmonary hypertension, atrial fibrillation, and pacemaker leads (**Table 1**). In these reports, approximately one-third of patients had a history of CAD, PCI, and CABG, however no granular data was available about the extent of RCA disease or the status of revascularization. Additionally, trans-catheter intervention reports do not include all patients developed TR after CABG as some of these patients may not be candidates for available trans-catheter trials. Thus, it would be difficult to estimate how many patients present with significant TR after CABG as this is not a common long-term outcome to study, which is primarily focused on survival and graft patency [12, 15, 16, 46, 47].

8. Conclusions

RV-free wall ischemic disease is not routinely addressed during the current CABG practice. The impact of ignoring the RV-free wall revascularization is not well examined in dedicated studies. In the early era of CABG evolution, there was more attention to RV-free wall ischemic disease; however, less attention continued toward RV revascularization. Due to the nature of the RV tolerance to ischemia and the presence of collateralization between the RCA and the left coronary system, the majority of patients with extended RCA disease may not have a prominent early impact of RV dysfunction if they underwent standard distal bypass. Perhaps this is the rationale for surgeons deviating away from RV-free wall revascularization in modern CABG practice, as they may not observe an early impact. However, the available data in the literature that we presented in this review suggests late RV dysfunction after CABG with worsening functional TR in some patients. This in part could be related to pulmonary hypertension or left-sided cardiac pathology, but it could also be very well related to ongoing RV-free wall ischemia that results in RV cardiomyopathy and functional TR, mimicking ischemic MR. At this point, further dedicated studies focusing on the long-term impact of ignoring RV-free wall ischemia are needed to develop a consensus, if proven significant. Addressing RV-free wall ischemic disease does not require additional complex procedures, but simply adding a bypass to an acute marginal branch or mid-RCA in patients with extended RCA disease (**Figure 1**). This may avoid the development of late RV dysfunction and functional TR in certain groups of patients with extended RCA disease without robust collateralization.

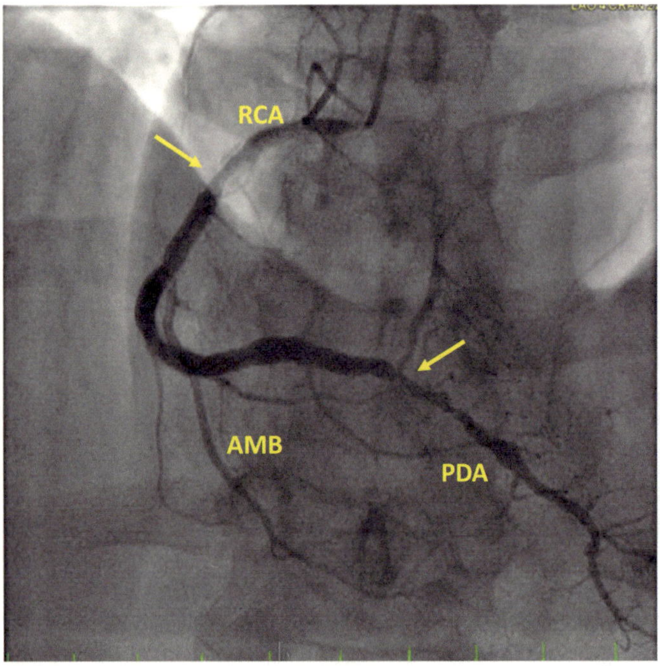

(a)

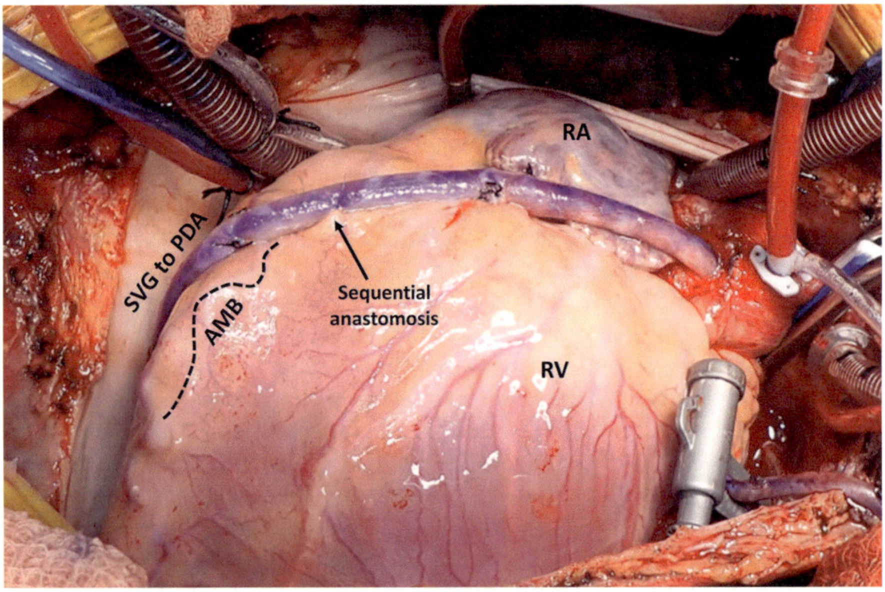

(b)

Figure 1.
A: Preoperative coronary angiogram showing significant in-stent stenosis lesion (arrow) of the proximal right coronary artery (RCA), significant lesion (arrow) in the proximal posterior descending artery (PDA), and a medium sized marginal artery branch (AMB) originating between the two lesions. B: Operative photo of bypass grafting to acute marginal branch (AMB, dashed line) using side-to-side sequential anastomosis technique (arrow) of the bypass graft to posterior descending artery (SVG to PDA). RA: Right atrium, RV: Right ventricle.

Conflict of interest

HE has financial relationship with Edwards Lifesciences, Artivion, and LifeNet Health. Rest of authors have nothing to disclose.

Author details

Haytham Elgharably[1*], Serge C. Harb[2], Amgad Mentias[2], Khaled Ziada[2] and Faisal G. Bakaeen[1]

1 Department of Thoracic and Cardiovascular Surgery, Cleveland Clinic Foundation, Heart and Vascular Institute, Cleveland, Ohio, United States

2 Department of Cardiovascular Medicine, Cleveland Clinic Foundation, Heart and Vascular Institute, Cleveland, Ohio, United States

*Address all correspondence to: elgharh@ccf.org

References

[1] Umana Pizano J, B, Arain FD, Harb SC, Bakaeen FG, Elgharably H. Is right ventricular free wall revascularization underrated? Sequential bypass of mid-right coronary artery to resolve acute right ventricular dysfunction. Journal of Thoracic and Cardiovascular Surgery Techniques. Oct 2023;**21**:118-121

[2] Bootsma IT, Scheeren TWL, de Lange F, Haenen J, Boonstra PW, Boerma EC. Impaired right ventricular ejection fraction after cardiac surgery is associated with a complicated ICU stay. Journal of Intensive Care. 2018;**6**:85

[3] Levy D, Laghlam D, Estagnasie P, Brusset A, Squara P, Nguyen LS. Post-operative right ventricular failure after cardiac surgery: A cohort study. Frontiers in Cardiovascular Medicine. 2021;**8**:667328

[4] Roshanali F, Yousefnia MA, Mandegar MH, Rayatzadeh H, Alinejad S. Decreased right ventricular function after coronary artery bypass grafting. Texas Heart Institute Journal. 2008;**35**:250-255

[5] Yadav H, Unsworth B, Fontana M, et al. Selective right ventricular impairment following coronary artery bypass graft surgery. European Journal of Cardio-Thoracic Surgery. 2010;**37**:393-398

[6] Chinikar M, Rafiee M, Aghajankhah M, et al. Right ventricular dysfunction and associated factors in patients after coronary artery bypass grafting. ARYA Atherosclerosis. 2019;**15**:99-105

[7] Elgharably H, Javadikasgari H, Koprivanac M, et al. Right versus left heart reverse remodelling after treating ischaemic mitral and tricuspid regurgitation. European Journal of Cardio-Thoracic Surgery. Feb 2021;**59**(2):442-450

[8] Ali, Sahin M, Yokuşoğlu M, Kuralay E, Ozal E. Can right ventricular branch bypass alleviate right ventricular dysfunction? Texas Heart Institute Journal. Sep 2022;**49**(5):e217607. DOI: 10.14503/THIJ-21-7607

[9] Güney MR, Eren E. Revascularization of multiple bypassable extended right coronary arteries. The Journal of Thoracic and Cardiovascular Surgery. 2004;**127**:1133-1138

[10] Ozerdem G, Katrancioglu N, Candemir B, Saricam E, Ozturk O, Berkan O. Effect of sequential coronary artery bypass venous grafting on right ventricular functions assessed by tissue Doppler echocardiography. Cardiovascular Journal of Africa. 2012;**23**:63-66

[11] Dimeling G, Bakaeen L, Khatri J, Bakaeen FG. CABG: When, why, and how? Cleveland Clinic Journal of Medicine. 2021;**88**:295-303

[12] McNichols B, Spratt JR, George J, Rizzi S, Manning EW, Park K. Coronary artery bypass: Review of surgical techniques and impact on long-term revascularization outcomes. Cardiology and Therapy. 2021;**10**:89-109

[13] Neumann FJ, Sousa-Uva M, Ahlsson A, et al. 2018 ESC/EACTS Guidelines on myocardial revascularization. European Heart Journal. 2019;**40**:87-165

[14] Lawton JS, Tamis-Holland JE, Bangalore S, et al. 2021 ACC/AHA/SCAI guideline for coronary artery revascularization: Executive summary:

A report of the American College of Cardiology/American Heart Association joint committee on clinical practice guidelines. Circulation. 2022;**145**:e4-e17

[15] Aldea GS, Bakaeen FG, Pal J, et al. The society of thoracic surgeons clinical practice guidelines on arterial conduits for coronary artery bypass grafting. The Annals of Thoracic Surgery. 2016;**101**:801-809

[16] Omer S, Cornwell LD, Rosengart TK, et al. Completeness of coronary revascularization and survival: Impact of age and off-pump surgery. The Journal of Thoracic and Cardiovascular Surgery. 2014;**148**:1307-15.e1

[17] Schwann TA, Yammine MB, El-Hage-Sleiman AM, Engoren MC, Bonnell MR, Habib RH. The effect of completeness of revascularization during CABG with single versus multiple arterial grafts. Journal of Cardiac Surgery. 2018;**33**:620-628

[18] Haddad F, Hunt SA, Rosenthal DN, Murphy DJ. Right ventricular function in cardiovascular disease, part I: Anatomy, physiology, aging, and functional assessment of the right ventricle. Circulation. 2008;**117**:1436-1448

[19] Rudski LG, Lai WW, Afilalo J, et al. Guidelines for the echocardiographic assessment of the right heart in adults: A report from the American society of echocardiography endorsed by the European association of echocardiography, a registered branch of the European society of cardiology, and the Canadian society of echocardiography. Journal of the American Society of Echocardiography: Official Publication of the American Society of Echocardiography. 2010;**23**:685-713; quiz 86-8

[20] Venkatachalam S, Wu G, Ahmad M. Echocardiographic assessment of the right ventricle in the current era: Application in clinical practice. Echocardiography (Mount Kisco, NY). 2017;**34**:1930-1947

[21] Bowers TR, O'Neill WW, Pica M, Goldstein JA. Patterns of coronary compromise resulting in acute right ventricular ischemic dysfunction. Circulation. 2002;**106**:1104-1109

[22] Lakatos B, Tősér Z, Tokodi M, et al. Quantification of the relative contribution of the different right ventricular wall motion components to right ventricular ejection fraction: The ReVISION method. Cardiovascular Ultrasound. 2017;**15**:8

[23] Kovács A, Lakatos B, Tokodi M, Merkely B. Right ventricular mechanical pattern in health and disease: Beyond longitudinal shortening. Heart Failure Reviews. 2019;**24**:511-520

[24] Vineberg A, Zamora B. Revascularization of the right ventricular myocardium via right coronary arterial system by right internal mammary artery implantation. The American Journal of Cardiology. 1968;**22**:218-226

[25] Rich JB, Akins CW, Daggett WM Jr. Right ventricular failure following cardiopulmonary bypass: Inadequate myocardial protection or incomplete revascularization? The Annals of Thoracic Surgery. 1988;**45**:693-694

[26] Cho S, Lee JH, Shim CY, et al. Abolished ischemic tricuspid regurgitation by revascularization of left anterior descending artery: The role of collateral circulation. Journal of Cardiology Cases. 2014;**10**:9-12

[27] Memic Sancar K, Topel C, Turen S, Erturk M, Babur Guler G. An overlooked cause for reversible severe tricuspid regurgitation and pulmonary

hypertension: Hibernating right ventricle. Echocardiography (Mount Kisco, NY). 2021;**38**:1450-1454

[28] Schofer J, Spielman R, Bleifeld W, Montz R, Mathey G. Scintigraphic evidence that the right ventricular myocardium tolerates ischaemia better than the left ventricular myocardium. European Heart Journal. 1985;**6**:751-758

[29] Navia JL, Elgharably H, Javadikasgari H, et al. Tricuspid regurgitation associated with ischemic mitral regurgitation: Characterization, evolution after mitral surgery, and value of tricuspid repair. The Annals of Thoracic Surgery. 2017;**104**:501-509

[30] Onorati F, Santarpino G, Marturano D, et al. Successful surgical treatment of chronic ischemic mitral regurgitation achieves left ventricular reverse remodeling but does not affect right ventricular function. The Journal of Thoracic and Cardiovascular Surgery. 2009;**138**:341-351

[31] De Bonis M, Lapenna E, Sorrentino F, et al. Evolution of tricuspid regurgitation after mitral valve repair for functional mitral regurgitation in dilated cardiomyopathy. European Journal of Cardio-Thoracic Surgery. 2008;**33**:600-606

[32] De Bonis M, Lapenna E, Pozzoli A, et al. Mitral valve repair without repair of moderate tricuspid regurgitation. The Annals of Thoracic Surgery. 2015;**100**:2206-2212

[33] Bertrand PB, Overbey JR, Zeng X, et al. Progression of tricuspid regurgitation after surgery for ischemic mitral regurgitation. Journal of the American College of Cardiology. 2021;**77**:713-724

[34] Koren O, Darawsha H, Rozner E, Benhamou D, Turgeman Y. Tricuspid regurgitation in ischemic mitral regurgitation patients: Prevalence, predictors for outcome and long-term follow-up. BMC Cardiovascular Disorders. 2021;**21**:199

[35] Elgharably H, Ibrahim A, Rosinski B, et al. Right heart failure and patient selection for isolated tricuspid valve surgery. The Journal of Thoracic and Cardiovascular Surgery. Sep 2023;**166**(3):740-751

[36] Alperi A, Almendárez M, Álvarez R, et al. Transcatheter tricuspid valve interventions: Current status and future perspectives. Frontiers in Cardiovascular Medicine. 2022;**9**:994502

[37] Besler C, Orban M, Rommel KP, et al. Predictors of procedural and clinical outcomes in patients with symptomatic tricuspid regurgitation undergoing transcatheter edge-to-edge repair. JACC Cardiovascular Interventions. 2018;**11**:1119-1128

[38] Fam NP, Braun D, von Bardeleben RS, et al. Compassionate use of the PASCAL transcatheter valve repair system for severe tricuspid regurgitation: A multicenter, observational, first-in-human experience. JACC Cardiovascular Interventions. 2019;**12**:2488-2495

[39] Kodali S, Hahn RT, Eleid MF, et al. Feasibility study of the transcatheter valve repair system for severe tricuspid regurgitation. Journal of the American College of Cardiology. 2021;**77**:345-356

[40] Nickenig G, Weber M, Schueler R, et al. 6-month outcomes of tricuspid valve reconstruction for patients with severe tricuspid regurgitation. Journal of the American College of Cardiology. 2019;**73**:1905-1915

[41] Davidson CJ, Lim DS, Smith RL, et al. Early feasibility study of cardioband

tricuspid system for functional tricuspid regurgitation: 30-day outcomes. JACC Cardiovascular Interventions. 2021;**14**:41-50

[42] Nickenig G, Friedrichs KP, Baldus S, et al. Thirty-day outcomes of the cardioband tricuspid system for patients with symptomatic functional tricuspid regurgitation: The TriBAND study. EuroIntervention: Journal of EuroPCR in Collaboration with the Working Group on Interventional Cardiology of the European Society of Cardiology. 2021;**17**:809-817

[43] Hahn RT, Meduri CU, Davidson CJ, et al. Early feasibility study of a transcatheter tricuspid valve annuloplasty: SCOUT trial 30-day results. Journal of the American College of Cardiology. 2017;**69**:1795-1806

[44] Hahn RT, Kodali S, Fam N, et al. Early multinational experience of transcatheter tricuspid valve replacement for treating severe tricuspid regurgitation. JACC Cardiovascular Interventions. 2020;**13**:2482-2493

[45] Fam NP, von Bardeleben RS, Hensey M, et al. Transfemoral transcatheter tricuspid valve replacement with the EVOQUE system: A multicenter, observational, first-in-human experience. JACC Cardiovascular Interventions. 2021;**14**:501-511

[46] Gaudino M, Samadashvili Z, Hameed I, Chikwe J, Girardi LN, Hannan EL. Differences in long-term outcomes after coronary artery bypass grafting using single vs multiple arterial grafts and the association with sex. JAMA Cardiology. 2020;**6**:401-409

[47] Hannan EL, Racz MJ, Walford G, et al. Long-term outcomes of coronary-artery bypass grafting versus stent implantation. The New England Journal of Medicine. 2005;**352**:2174-2183

Chapter 5

Overview of Coronary Artery Bypass Surgery

Jorge Balaguer and Leshya Bokka

Abstract

This chapter provides an overview of coronary artery bypass surgery in clinical practice, beginning with a discussion about implications from a public health perspective, followed by indications for coronary artery bypass grafting (CABG), surgical options in heart failure patients, and minimally invasive approaches. Specific areas discussed include on- versus off-pump CABG, robotic procedures, coronary endarterectomy, the Dor procedure (Surgical Ventricular Restoration), Impella® and Intra-aortic balloon pump (IABP)-supported CABG, trans-myocardial laser revascularization (TMR), and hybrid and multiple arterial revascularization techniques. To conclude is a discussion on the growing importance of surgical simulation and different models of simulators in training residents and fellows. Faculty members similarly benefit from surgical simulation, particularly for complex or less frequent revascularization procedures.

Keywords: robotic procedures, simulation, public health, indications, heart failure patients, education, overview

1. Introduction

The first planned coronary artery bypass graft (CABG) operation, intended to treat chronic coronary artery disease (CAD), was performed by Dr. René Favaloro at the Cleveland Clinic in 1967 [1]. This initial procedure involved anastomosing a saphenous vein graft (SVG) from the proximal right coronary artery (RCA) to the distal RCA. Soon after, the technique evolved into performing the proximal anastomosis to the ascending aorta and became known as aorto-coronary bypass. Since its introduction, several improvements have been very impactful and widely adopted. Of note is the comparison between CABG and the less-invasive revascularization option, percutaneous coronary intervention (PCI), as a means for myocardial revascularization due to coronary artery disease (CAD). As PCI techniques and technology developed significantly over the last decades, this option gained popularity due to increased accessibility and advances in drug-eluting stent technology (DES). CABG is still the preferred revascularization intervention for patients with advanced CAD and remains the gold standard treatment for coronary revascularization, particularly in some subsets of patients, showing superior outcomes compared to PCI/stenting and guideline-directed medical therapy (GDMT) in patients with advanced CAD. This chapter outlines the indications for CABG and its public health implications and considerations for special populations.

IntechOpen

2. Epidemiology and public health

CAD is the leading cause of mortality globally, accounting for 17.9 million deaths [2]. The leading symptom of CAD is angina, which could lead to different types of myocardial infarctions, ventricular arrhythmias, and heart failure. CAD significantly impacts quality of life as well as life expectancy and disability. Ischemic cardiomyopathy is responsible for about half of heart failure cases in the United States. Patients from low- and middle-income countries have a high disease burden from delayed presentation and treatment secondary to advanced disease, poor healthcare services access, and delayed treatments, resulting in excess mortality. In the United States, cardiovascular disease accounts for over $300 billion annually, and ischemic heart disease spending was just under $80 billion [3].

Despite the World Health Organization's targets to decrease morbidity and mortality from non-communicable diseases, CAD and stroke deaths are rising in the United States [4]. CABG is the most frequently performed cardiac operation, with about 400,000 CABG operations being performed each year in the United States [5, 6]. Overall, CAD contributes to significant morbidity and mortality globally, and coronary revascularization offers the chance for myocardial recovery. Coronary revascularization offers an incredibly effective treatment for myocardial function and protection that offers improved survival and event-free survival. CABG is a robust palliative intervention as the healthcare community and major public health organizations work towards enhancing primary prevention interventions targeting the incidence of CAD.

3. Indications for CABG

In the last decade, the SYNergy between percutaneous coronary intervention with TAXus and cardiac surgery (SYNTAX) score became a widely used, accurate method to objectively assess the severity of CAD. Used for the first time in the SYNTAX Trial, the SYNTAX score is a valuable tool to aid clinicians in deciding the best strategy for revascularization [7]. A high SYNTAX score reflects a high burden of CAD; these patients greatly benefit from CABG if the surgical risk is low or moderate. Considering that some patients with advanced CAD are elderly, frail, or may have a significant degree of cardiac and non-cardiac comorbidities, the decision to proceed with CABG must account for the risk of morbidity and mortality associated with such an operation. Risk stratification models, including the Society for Thoracic Surgeons (STS), EuroScore, and many others, aid surgeons and heart teams in this decision-making process [8].

CABG and PCI are the two direct revascularization options used today. Both interventions are very effective and have been part of clinical practice for decades. Multiple studies have evaluated the benefit of each procedure in specific patient populations. CABG is the best intervention in patients with left main disease, three-vessel CAD, diabetes, and high SYNTAX scores [9, 10]. Mortality rates for emergency CABG and reoperations are high, likely due to severe illness and higher acuity at presentation. Alternatives to CABG are usually explored in these cases. In patients with three-vessel CAD or two-vessel CAD with proximal left anterior descending (LAD) artery involvement, CABG is a superior option, mainly based on the benefits of grafting the LAD with the left internal mammary artery (LIMA).

In contrast, PCI is the preferred intervention if the LAD is not involved [9, 10]. CABG outperformed GDMT in patients with advanced CAD, particularly if the

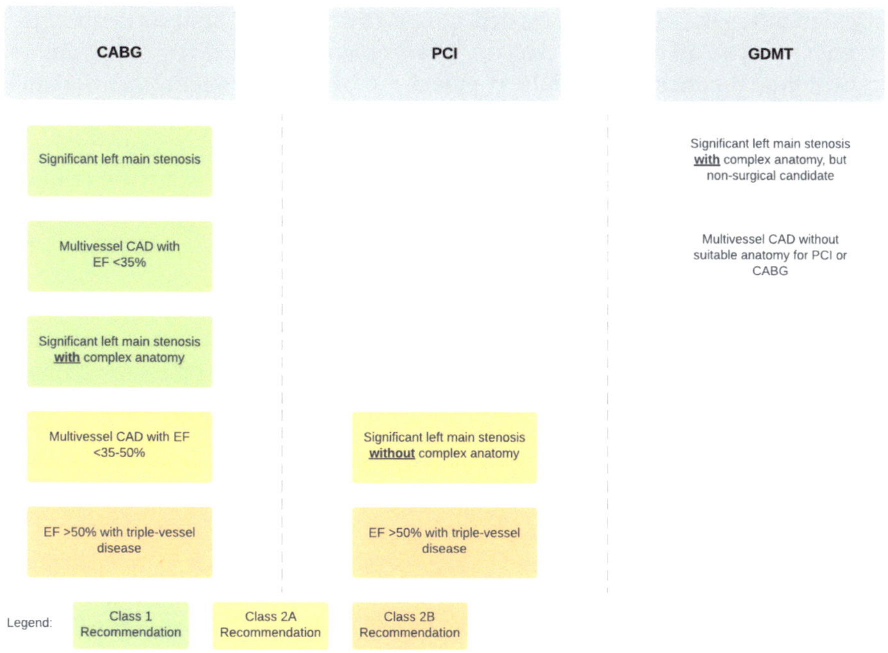

Figure 1.
American Heart Association recommendations for the management of stable ischemic heart disease (SIHD) in patients with angina refractory to medical therapy [9].

LAD is involved [11, 12]. While PCI is preferred over surgical intervention for AMI, cardiac surgery remains the primary mode of intervention for complications of AMI, including free wall ventricular rupture, ventricular septal rupture (VSR), and acute mitral insufficiency secondary to papillary muscle rupture. In these cases, the goal of care is two-fold: revascularizing myocardium and repairing post-infarct mechanical complications.

For patients with multi-vessel disease and ischemic cardiomyopathy with an ejection fraction (EF) < 35%, CABG is the preferred surgical approach, offering increased survival and symptom relief (**Figure 1**) [9, 11].

4. Interventions

Although the fundamentals of surgical revascularization have changed very little since its introduction, multiple improvements have led to safer, less invasive operations with shorter recovery times. Surgical revascularization provides higher value if performed in higher-risk and more complex patient populations. Several approaches are now available for surgical coronary artery revascularization. This section outlines the traditional CABG operation, minimally invasive options, ventricular restoration considerations, coronary endarterectomies, and trans-myocardial laser revascularization.

4.1 General approach

The basic principle behind the CABG operation involves constructing arterial and venous grafts to improve blood supply distal to the site of a coronary obstruction.

Revascularization in CABG requires delicate microvascular techniques in order to anastomose very small coronary arteries (1 to 2 mm in diameter) to grafts using very delicate monofilament sutures (Polypropylene 7-0 or 8-0), thinner than a human hair. The core surgical steps of the traditional CABG surgery include performing a median sternotomy, establishing access for cardiopulmonary bypass (CPB), and arresting the heart to obtain a motionless surgical field. Once these critical steps are achieved, arterial and venous vessel grafting can be performed (**Figures 2** and **3**).

Considerations for choosing "target vessels" for grafting to the coronary arteries include carefully analyzing multimodal anatomic factors of the coronary arteries to be bypassed. The coronary arteriogram is the gold standard, state-of-the-art imaging to evaluate the severity of lesions and site to perform distal anastomosis to the surgical target. The use of Intravascular Ultrasound (IVUS) and Functional Flow Reserve (FFR) assist in identifying significant lesions when images from the coronary arteriogram are not definitive. The graft choice is critical and should be individualized for each patient. These considerations make CABG a "tailor-made operation" designed specifically for each patient. Arterial grafts have demonstrated superior patency than venous grafts for multiple biologic factors; however, arterial grafts can be vulnerable to competitive flow and vasoconstriction, described in radial arterial grafts as the "string sign." The use of the LIMA is universally accepted and is utilized on most patients undergoing CABG where the LAD must be bypassed. The LIMA-to-LAD anastomosis has shown increased survival and decreased major adverse cardiovascular events. The additive value of using a second or a third arterial graft is less established when its risks are considered. Other factors such as diabetes, patient's age, life expectancy, and lesion severity must be assessed before proceeding with multi-arterial revascularization.

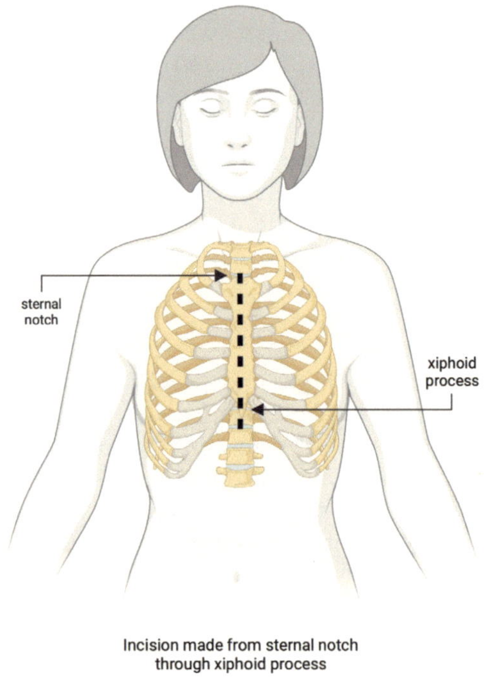

Figure 2.
Median sternotomy incision.

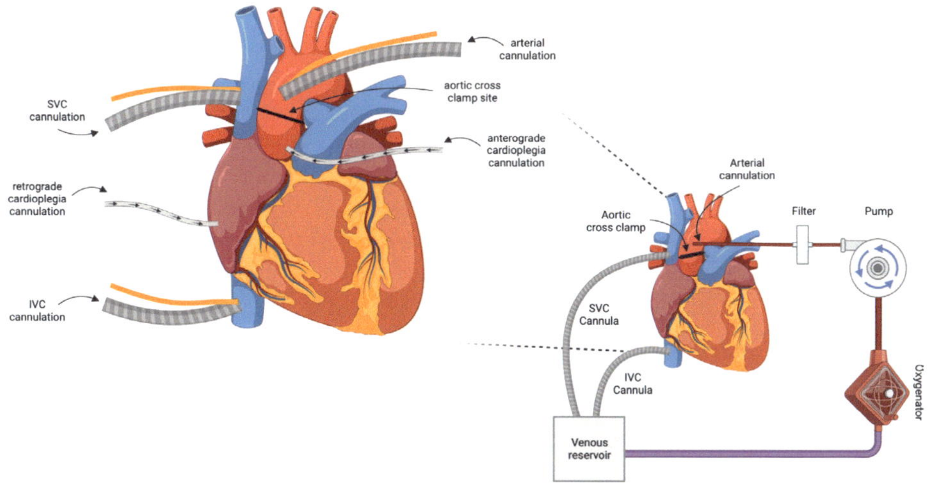

Figure 3.
Cannulation for cardiopulmonary bypass and flow of blood through cardiopulmonary bypass pump.

Strictly from the vascular behaviors of individual grafts, arterial grafts have demonstrated higher patency when compared to SVG. While LIMA grafts have a patency of over 90% beyond the 10-year mark [13, 14], SVG grafts have failure rates between 15% and up to 25% within the first 18 months [15]. Approximately 50% of all vein grafts become diseased, and many become occluded 10 years after CABG due to vein graft CAD, which results from a combination of early endothelial damage during surgery, inflammation, and gradual lipid deposition [16]. The more extensive use of arterial grafts is appealing, as they are protected from the biological failure seen on vein grafts; however, care should be taken when using the RIMA and the radial artery. The use of multiple arterial grafts may pose additional risks and may not significantly benefit the patient. Sternal complications are of concern when using the LIMA and the right internal mammary artery (RIMA) in the same patient [17]. Harvesting the internal mammary artery compromises sternal blood flow [17, 18]. Using the LIMA and RIMA simultaneously significantly decreases sternal blood flow, compromising sternal wound healing and increasing the risk of sternal complications, including infection [17]. The effect of poor sternal wound healing is more pronounced in patients with diabetes. Skeletonizing the LIMA and RIMA involves harvesting only the arteries without their associated veins or fascia, which mitigates this risk (**Figure 4**) [19].

Vasospasm and string sign due to competitive flow in radial artery grafts is infrequent if the target vessel being bypassed has more than 70% stenosis, and even lower if the stenosis is above 90%. Biological factors that influence venous graft patency are endothelial damage and low levels of arterial endothelial cell factors, including nitric oxide, that help decrease inflammation and thrombosis. The coronary system where the anastomosis is performed also affects patency. The LIMA-to-LAD anastomosis is favorable due to the position of both vessels (LIMA and LAD) and the extensive run-off of the LAD system. Coronary artery diameter also influences patency. The larger the coronary artery, the better the patency, independent of the graft used.

Patient comorbidities also guide graft selection. For example, patients with chronic kidney disease (CKD) may not be suitable candidates for radial artery grafting to preserve the radial artery in case of fistula placement. In addition, the radial

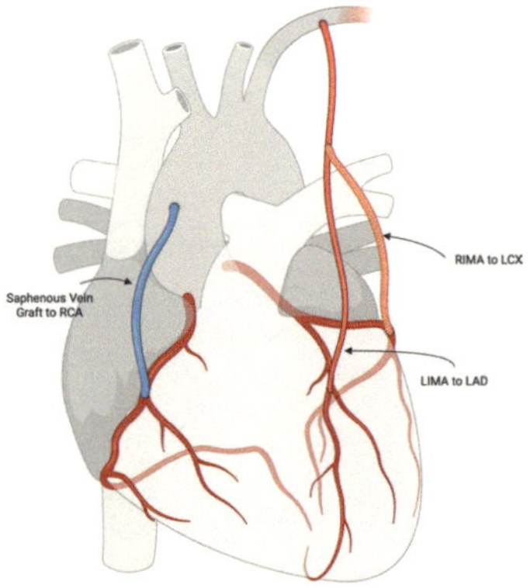

Figure 4.
Multi-arterial grafting.

artery is unsuitable in patients with insufficient ulnar artery flow, as grafting the radial artery will compromise hand perfusion, although this is an infrequent event. Patients with advanced vascular disease may have poor radial artery quality as well. If the patient had a recent cardiac catheterization via the radial artery, this vessel should not be used for grafting. Preoperative ultrasound of the radial artery, ulnar artery, and patency of palmar arches are evaluated prior to using the radial artery as a graft.

4.2 Minimally invasive CABG

Less invasive approaches to traditional CABG operations via median sternotomy and extracorporeal circulation were introduced to clinical practice in the 1990s. The first iteration of a minimally invasive direct CABG (MIDCAB) involved minimizing the surgical trauma associated with a traditional CABG. MIDCAB (minimally invasive direct coronary artery bypass) is sought after for several reasons. While a traditional CABG allows for complete visualization of the heart in an immobile and blood-free operative field, it requires several invasive steps, including a median sternotomy that divides the sternum, cannulation CPB via the ascending aorta (most common), and cardioplegic arrest. The alternatives described are intended to avoid these complex and potentially risky steps to minimize surgical trauma, decrease surgical morbidity, and enhance recovery. This section outlines the advantages and disadvantages of these alternative approaches.

Sources of morbidity associated with traditional CABG operation come from three main steps: (1) median sternotomy, (2) CPB, and (3) cardioplegic arrest. The median sternotomy of a traditional CABG is performed as an incision dividing the sternum longitudinally. One or both halves of the sternum get de-vascularized in the process. Approximately 30–40% of patients subjected to CABG operations are diabetics. In addition to diabetes, comorbidities such as COPD and obesity increase the risk of sternal complications, including osteomyelitis, acute mediastinitis, and poor wound healing. While these complications are uncommon (1%), they are serious, morbid conditions.

Performing a CABG through a small 8 cm incision on the left side of the chest became the first step to reducing the mechanical trauma to the chest wall. In MIDCAB, the risk of sternal complications is of low concern due to the sternum being left intact. Similarly, mini-thoracotomy and limited anterior thoracotomy are both approaches to decrease the stress from sternal devascularization and rib spreading. Fewer and smaller incisions also aid in post-operative wound healing and decrease the risk of wound infections. Micro-fixation systems, including titanium plates and screws, help reduce wound healing complications, especially in those with high-risk comorbidities, and enhances bone healing [20, 21].

The physiologic impact of CPB has been extensively documented; it involves artificial, non-pulsatile perfusion, resulting in the potential for whole-body inflammatory response, endothelial damage, and end-organ damage, particularly in patients with pre-existing or underlying cerebrovascular disease, visceral disease, and renal dysfunction. The mechanical stress cells undergo while contacting the extracorporeal circulation surface is another source of the inflammatory process, which has been well confirmed with an increase of other serum pro-inflammatory markers [22–24]. Total body inflammatory response leads to vasoplegia, coagulopathy, third spacing, platelet activation, and subsequent platelet dysfunction [22–24]. In addition, CPB cannulation induces the risk of disrupting atherosclerotic plaques in the ascending aorta (common in older patients), which is directly associated with intraoperative embolic stroke with devastating consequences [25, 26].

An alternative approach is to perform CABG without CPB, which mitigates the physiologic disarray that takes place when the patient's blood encounters the inner surface of the extracorporeal circulation tubing. This method is known as off-pump CABG (OPCAB). Depending on the situation, MIDCAB could also be performed with extracorporeal circulation via cannulation of the femoral vessels while still limiting chest wall trauma.

Lastly, in traditional CABG, cardioplegic arrest is necessary to operate on an arrested heart. This step is essentially a controlled ischemic event to which the myocardium is subjected. Patients with depressed ventricular function are more vulnerable to complications of cardioplegic arrest, including intra- and post-operative systolic and diastolic dysfunction. Despite using state-of-the-art myocardial protection solutions, consequences could include worsened ventricular dysfunction and cardiogenic shock (**Table 1**).

4.2.1 On- vs. off-pump

In patients with pre-existing aortic atherosclerosis, chronic kidney disease, cerebrovascular disease, visceral vascular disease, liver cirrhosis, bone marrow suppression, and diabetes, CPB may pose a higher risk of end-organ dysfunction and stroke. OPCAB, or beating heart CABG, is an attractive surgical option in such patients. OPCAB still requires a traditional median sternotomy, and because CPB and cardioplegia are not used during this approach, OPCAB confers the advantage of reduced inflammatory response, lower risk of end-organ dysfunction, and lower risk and stroke. However, as expected, anastomoses are technically more challenging in an OPCAB, particularly in visualizing the lateral wall. Regional ischemia while the anastomosis is being performed and dysfunction can occur. In expert hands, OPCAB produces comparable revascularization to traditional on-pump CABG, lower perioperative morbidity, particularly regarding stroke, and excellent long-term results.

4.2.2 Minimally invasive direct CABG (MIDCAB)

Minimally invasive direct coronary artery bypass (MIDCAB) involves a small thoracic incision in the left fourth or fifth intercostal space to harvest the LIMA and perform

Traditional CABG vs. minimally invasive options

Technique	Traditional median sternotomy	Cardiopulmonary Bypass	Cardioplegic Arrest	Proximal anastomosis to aorta	Advantages	Disadvantages
Traditional CABG	X	X	X	X	• Unobstructed view	• Wound healing • Inflammation
OPCAB	X			X	• Reduced inflammatory response	• Myocardial motion • Limited surgical view, especially of posterior and lateral regions • Regional ischemia during anastomosis
MIDCAB			+/–		• Small thoracic incisions that may not require rib spreading	• Difficult to access PDA and distal RCA • Technically difficult graft harvesting
MVST CABG		+/–			• Small anterior thoracotomy	• Limited access

OPCAB = off-pump coronary artery bypass graft; MIDCAB = minimally invasive direct coronary artery bypass graft; MVST CABG = multivessel small thoracotomy coronary artery bypass graft; and +/– indicates can be performed either with or without.

Table 1.
Comparison of minimally invasive CABG techniques.

an off-pump LIMA-to-LAD anastomosis. The LIMA is harvested through the small incision as far superiorly as possible, usually with specialized instruments and equipment. Stabilization devices may allow for more precise anastomosis of the LIMA to the LAD. In some cases, and in expert hands, more extensive revascularization may be performed by accessing the ascending aorta to perform proximal anastomoses as required.

MIDCAB offers the double benefit of reduced thoracic trauma and avoiding extracorporeal circulation and its inflammatory response, leading to faster recovery times and shorter hospital lengths of stay. However, this approach is technically demanding.

Multivessel small thoracotomy (MVST) and minimally invasive coronary surgery (MICS) share the same principles of MIDCAB and can be considered a subcategory of MIDCAB. However, as the name suggests, MVST CABG allows multiple anastomoses to be performed on various coronary vessels. Commonly used grafts include the LIMA and radial artery. MIDCAB, MVST CABG, and MICS are technically demanding operations with steep learning curves. These procedures are considered expert operations and should be performed at centers with highly experienced and skilled teams.

4.2.3 Robotic procedures

It has been decades since the Da Vinci Robot was introduced to the field of cardiac surgery. Robotic cases have been mainly directed towards mitral valve and coronary operations. Outstanding advancements in tools have enhanced the possibilities of coronary surgery. For example, the endo-wrist allows improved maneuvering that exceeds a surgeon's inherent hand mobility. Features such as enhanced visualization and three-dimensional optics offer 10X image magnification, thus, providing superior conditions for surgical performance. Despite these capabilities, acquiring expertise in robotic procedures is associated with a steep learning curve. As a result, robotic procedures have been adopted relatively slowly, particularly in coronary surgery.

In expert hands, the outcomes of Totally Endoscopic Coronary Artery Bypass (TECAB) are impressive, providing complete, all arterial revascularization using LIMA and RIMA using only port sites and mostly performed off-pump [27]. Anastomoses are performed on a closed chest using anastomotic connectors [28–32] or are sewn using robotic arms. Patients may be safely discharged 24–48 hours postoperatively because this operation is associated with minimal surgical trauma (chest wall and physiologic trauma). A common alternative to the TECAB is the Robotic Assisted MIDCAB [27, 33, 34]. With the assistance of the Da Vinci Robot, the LIMA is harvested with minimal rib spreading. Then, a small incision (4 cm is performed in the 4th or 5th LICS to identify the LAD. Under direct vision, the LIMA-LAD anastomosis is then performed off-pump.

Robotic approaches are ideal for patients with CAD limited to the LAD or proximal LAD, although more extensive revascularization can be performed in expert hands [27]. Hybrid revascularization considerations are becoming more popular for patients with two- or three-vessel CAD interested in a minimally invasive approach for the LIMA-to-LAD anastomosis while utilizing third-generation DES for the remainder of the affected non-LAD coronary vessels. This option allows for the long-term benefits of bypass surgery while minimizing the trauma of a median sternotomy.

4.2.4 Hybrid revascularization procedures

Considering that the LIMA-to-LAD is the most critical graft in a CABG operation. This graft is primarily responsible for increased survival and low rates of MACCE;

therefore, it would be reasonable to propose that a minimally invasive LIMA-to-LAD (MIDCAB, robot-assisted MIDCAB or TECAB) combined with stenting of the circumflex and RCA systems with third-generation DES would lead to the "best of both worlds" [35]. Complete revascularization with the combination of LIMA and DES would be achieved with minimal trauma [35]. Intraoperative angiography would also be performed to confirm the quality of the LIMA-to-LAD anastomosis while the patient is still in the operating room, provided that the operation takes place in a hybrid operating room [35]. Using such approaches allows the surgeon to confirm complete revascularization [35]. Patients undergoing this hybrid procedure have enhanced recovery, spend only 2 or 3 days in the hospital, are able to drive in 10–14 days, and return to unrestricted activity in three to 4 weeks. Several studies have validated the benefits of this approach [36]. Third- and fourth-generation stents are demonstrating comparable results with respect to graft patency compared to vein grafts [37]. By contrast, no current stent has been shown to be superior to the LIMA-to-LAD anastomosis, supporting the use of a hybrid approach. These indisputable results support the use of a hybrid approach for revascularization.

4.2.5 IABP and Impella® supported CABG

Intra-aortic balloon pump (IABP) and Impella ®-supported CABG are practical approaches utilized to assist the left ventricle function and overall hemodynamics in patients with ischemic cardiomyopathy (ejection fraction (EF) < 30%) who require surgical revascularization. Patients with advanced CAD and heart failure frequently have a depressed EF. The etiology of low EF varies from infarcted to hibernating myocardium (chronically ischemic but alive). Infarcted myocardium will not recover its function after revascularization while hibernating myocardium will. Patients with depressed EF are a high-risk surgical population that would greatly benefit from coronary surgery [9, 10, 38]. These benefits were more recently confirmed by a 10-year follow-up study of the original Surgical Treatment for Ischemic Heart Failure (STICH) trial, in which the advantages of surgery over medical management, particularly in terms of survival, is demonstrated with statistical significance [39].

One of the challenges with these patients is the perioperative management and the risk of postoperative cardiogenic shock. For many years, patients in this group underwent IABP-supported CABG, which involved placing an IABP 24–48 hours before surgery. The IABP remains in place postoperatively for the necessary length of time until signs of hemodynamic and ventricular function improvement and stunned myocardium resolution, generally a few days. Although helpful, the disadvantages of this approach are reflected by the need for prolonged bedrest, leading to physical deconditioning and lower extremity muscle weakness. In addition, peripheral vascular complications involving the lower extremities are complications of IABP via the femoral arteries, particularly left in situ for several days. It is essential to mention that the IABP does provide a moderate increase in cardiac output and blood pressure while decreasing afterload. However, one of its limitations is that it does not decompress the left ventricle meaningfully, especially when compared to the Impella® device.

More recently, since the introduction of Impella® [40], many patients with low EF and heart failure have undergone bypass surgery supported by Impella® instead of an IABP. The Impella® device, available in varying sizes and power, is placed into the left ventricular cavity and ascending aorta across the aortic valve via femoral, axillary/subclavian, or ascending aorta [41]. The Impella® device has an inlet pump that draws in blood from the LV. This blood then moves through the device and, via a sophisticated intra-corporeal pump, is pumped out distal to the aortic valve on the ascending aorta.

In addition to the ventricular support during CABG, decompression of the left ventricle with the Impella® is highly beneficial and decreases the left ventricular diameter, reducing oxygen consumption by reducing myocardial oxygen demand [41]. The 5.5 model of the Impella® pump has the ability to pump up to 5 L per minute, providing superior hemodynamic support and increasing coronary artery and end-organ perfusion [40]. As a result, these patients can be out of bed by postoperative day one and ambulate while the Impella® remains in place. In other words, as the device is being weaned, the patient is already eating, ambulating, and undergoing physical rehabilitation. The Impella® device is removed at the bedside under local anesthesia as the myocardium stunning recovers between days four and seven.

Many surgical groups, including ours, favor using the Impella® device in this capacity for patients with severely decreased ventricular function, more advanced cardiomyopathy, and heart failure.

4.3 Coronary endarterectomy

Coronary endarterectomy (CE) was the mainstay for coronary artery revascularization prior to CABG. CE refers to stripping atherosclerotic plaque of extended length from a diseased coronary artery and therefore recreating the lumen of the vessel. Due to the complexity of CE, it is more demanding than CABG, and it is often only performed alongside CABG. Age, advanced CAD, and comorbidities such as diabetes or hyperlipidemia may increase the rate of more diffuse CAD and the need for CE. The presence of diabetes is especially notable for associations with diffuse CAD. In the current era, CE is rarely performed but it might constitute the only option to achieve myocardial revascularization.

Considerations for maintaining the patency of the coronary vessels after CE include maintaining some degree of anticoagulation in the postoperative period. As soon as surgical bleeding is not an issue, postoperative dual antiplatelet therapy with aspirin + clopidogrel or aspirin + ticagrelor will assist in mitigating the risk of early thrombosis. Some surgeons may decide to only partially reverse heparinization in the OR to maintain some early anticoagulation and prevent thrombosis.

The procedure itself involves creating a small proximal arteriotomy in the diseased coronary vessel. Then, a plane between the tunica media and atherosclerotic plaque is established via blunt and sharp dissection to begin the process of releasing plaque from the vessel. The endarterectomized coronary artery is grafted appropriately with a patch or directly with a graft. In addition, intraoperative angiography can be used in conjunction with hybrid operating rooms to verify the completion of CE and graft patency.

CE has higher postoperative morbidity compared to CABG alone [42, 43], but both short- and long-term patency have been demonstrated in CE in combination with CABG [44, 45]. MI rates are up to 10% [46, 47]. Despite the higher risk of perioperative complications associated with CE, it is essential to consider that these patients present with more advanced, diffuse CAD and calcified vessels, posing a higher perioperative risk regardless of whether CE is performed (**Figure 5**).

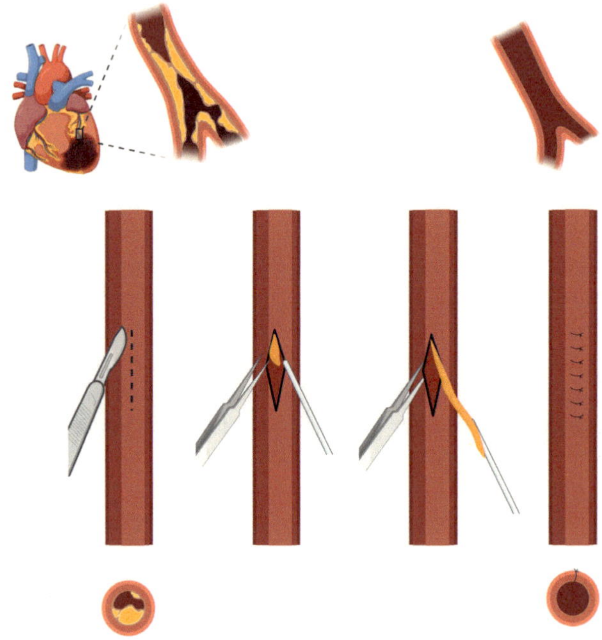

Figure 5.
Coronary endarterectomy.

4.3.1 Other revascularization techniques

Trans-myocardial laser revascularization (TMR) employs the energy of a laser to create channels from the epicardium to the endocardium, where areas of ischemic myocardium are identified by nuclear test and by coronary artery disease substrate. Lasers employ carbon dioxide or holmium yttrium-aluminum-garnett to induce angiogenesis in the treated areas to mitigate the decreased blood supply in treated myocardial regions. TMR involves performing a left anterolateral thoracotomy through which the ischemic myocardium is treated via laser pulses of energy delivered during ventricular diastole. This operation is performed off-pump. No heparinization is required.

Studies have shown a significant decrease in angina symptoms [48–52] but no survival benefits after TMR [51, 53]. While there was an improvement in angina symptoms, it is difficult to document directly improved perfusion in treated areas. These findings suggest that the mechanism by which TMR produces a therapeutic effect of angina relief has yet to be precisely identified. As with traditional CE, TMR may be used concomitantly with CABG to improve the revascularization of distally diseased vessels.

Indications for TMR as a sole therapy include patients with Canadian class III/IV angina symptoms for whom direct revascularization via PCI or CABG is not feasible [48, 54, 55]. Nuclear imaging studies should be obtained to evaluate for ischemic myocardium. Patients without angina, with an EF <30%, unstable angina, and without ischemia on thallium stress tests are not candidates for TMR. When combined with CABG, TMR has shown clear benefits in short-term survival [56]. Coronary targets amenable to CABG should be grafted. Territories with poor-quality arteries not amenable to grafting or stenting should be considered for laser revascularization in combination with CABG (**Figure 6**).

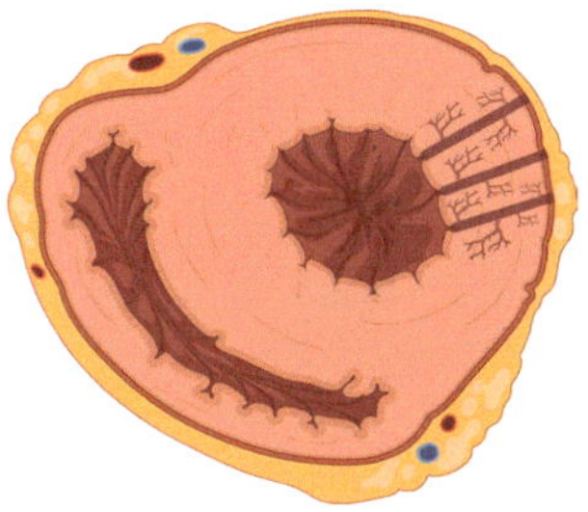

Figure 6.
Angiogenesis surrounding channels created by CO2 laser in TMR.

5. Surgical ventricular restoration (SVR) (Dor procedure)

Although SVR, also called the Dor procedure, is not a revascularization procedure per se, coronary surgeons are frequently consulted for patients with ischemic cardiomyopathy with a low EF. It is common to evaluate patients with a dyskinetic or akinetic apex, anterior wall, or distal septum after a STEMI involving the LAD. Frequently, isolated left ventricular dysfunction occurs.

Left ventricular remodeling is responsible for left ventricular dilatation, which is quantified by left ventricular end-diastolic volume (LVEDV), left ventricular end-systolic volume (LVESV), left ventricular end-diastolic diameter (LVEDD), left ventricular end-systolic diameter (LVESD), and the corresponding indices. In ischemic cardiomyopathy with low EF, these measures demonstrate a dilated, ineffective left ventricle. Congestive heart failure, low cardiac output, and ventricular arrhythmias are common sequelae of left ventricular remodeling.

Patients with ischemic cardiomyopathy with depressed EF benefit from surgical revascularization of viable territories in addition to the removal of the infarcted area and surgical ventricular restoration. The affected area may be aneurysmal. SVR decreases ventricular volume and increases EF, making the left ventricle more conical in shape and efficient, as the viable myocardium is revascularized. SVR is different from LV aneurysm repair, but both are operations that fall under the category of ventricular volume reduction operations. These techniques are frequently combined with the IABP and Impella® devices for hemodynamic support in the perioperative period. The STICH trial compared CABG + SVR vs. CABG alone [57]. Although this study showed no differences between these two techniques [57], in expert hands, patients undergoing CABG + SVR have improved, event-free survival (**Figure 7**).

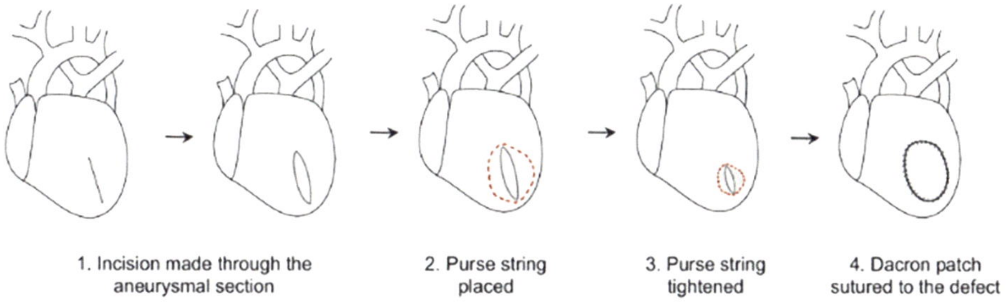

Figure 7.
The Dor procedure.

6. Diabetic patients

Since hypothesis-generated data emerged from the Bypass Angioplasty Revascularization Investigation (BARI) trial [58], CABG has been the preferred revascularization approach in diabetic patients with advanced CAD. Approximately 40% of all patients undergoing coronary revascularization have diabetes [59]. Rates of arteriolosclerosis are higher among diabetic patients because of the nature of the disease (proliferation, inflammation) and the prothrombotic nature of diabetes. As a result, diabetic patients are more likely to have complex, multivessel CAD involving large territories of the myocardium. Both the Future REvascularization Evaluation in patients with Diabetes Mellitus (FREEDOM) and SYNTAX trials found CABG to outperform PCI in this patient population [7, 60, 61]. The Bypass Angioplasty Revascularization Investigation 2 Diabetes (BARI 2D) trial found reduced cardiovascular events with CABG compared to GDMT [62]. Higher rates of repeat revascularization were found in diabetic patients who initially underwent PCI. Overall, diabetic patients experience higher mortality and cardiovascular complications when treated with PCI [63]. This finding can be partially explained by the diffuse nature of CAD in diabetic patients, making CABG a better intervention to achieve complete revascularization.

Diabetic patients are also prone to wound infection, impaired wound healing, and renal complications [7, 64]. In terms of the approach for CABG, bilateral IMA grafting is very selectively recommended due to high rates of wound infection. In summary, the SYNTAX, BARI 2D, and FREEDOM trials support CABG for diabetic patients with multivessel CAD [7, 60, 62]; CABG is associated with better outcomes, as the underlying disease pathophysiology is more extensive. In addition, a more complete revascularization is obtained via CABG, resulting in better outcomes. Capitalizing on the LIMA-to-LAD anastomosis is critical in reaping the benefits of CABG in diabetic patients.

7. Simulation training

Simulation has assumed a more significant role in medical education and surgical training. An exceptionally high level of expertise and skill is required to perform the previously discussed complex coronary operations. An increasing number of general surgery and cardiothoracic surgery training programs have incorporated surgical simulations of various modalities into their programs. Wet labs, virtual reality platforms, robotic training, and didactics are central to enhancing the trainees' technical skills and clinical knowledge before progressing to surgery in the clinical realm. Senior cardiac surgeons, professors, and mentors are key elements in this process.

The benefits of simulation training are widely documented, as there is no risk to patient safety, and learners are allowed to practice high-acuity, technically demanding procedures in a safe yet controlled environment. Simulation enables learners to practice technical skills unique to cardiac surgery while gaining direct exposure to and an appreciation for the art of cardiac surgery. More recent literature is now showing how simulation training modalities increased engagement with and knowledge of cardiac surgery procedures [65]. A high faculty-to-learner ratio and hands-on experiences were among some of the factors that contributed to learner satisfaction with simulation training [65].

Increasing exposure to cardiac operations early in training via simulation education is vital in increasing interest in and engagement with cardiac surgery as a field. Studies suggest cardiac surgeons choose subspecialty early in residency, if not in medical school. Medical students and junior residents are the ideal target population for recruiting future cardiac surgeons.

8. Conclusions

Coronary artery revascularization has experienced significant improvements since the first CABG was performed. The advent of PCI and DES have significantly contributed to the interventional care of patients with CAD. However, CABG remains the preferred revascularization technique for patients with advanced CAD.

The LIMA-to-LAD graft and the completeness of revascularization (not affected by the SYNTAX Score) are highly responsible for most of the long-term benefits of CABG. As the field of coronary surgery moves into the era of minimally invasive approaches, MIDCAB, MICS, robotic cardiac surgery, and OPCAB offer less invasive options to minimize the morbidity associated with traditional on-pump, trans-sternal CABG while preserving the benefits of the traditional operation. Using the RIMA and radial arteries as additional arterial grafts, as opposed to saphenous veins, in addition to the LIMA, extends the long-term benefits of bypass surgery.

Coronary endarterectomy and TMR complement the final treatment of the patients who are screened for CABG. Operations that treat the sequela of ischemic heart disease, including SVR (Dor Procedure) and LV aneurysm repair, are valuable surgical options for patients with ischemic cardiomyopathy. Mechanical complications of STEMI still require repair of the underlying mechanical problem, such as interventricular septal rupture, ventricular free wall rupture, and acute mitral regurgitation secondary to papillary muscle rupture. Multimodal simulation allows trainees and experienced surgeons to train for high-complexity coronary operations, minimally invasive approaches, and other high-acuity operations without compromising patient safety.

Acknowledgements

Figures 2–6 created with BioRender.com.

Conflict of interest

The authors declare no conflict of interest.

Author details

Jorge Balaguer[1] and Leshya Bokka[2*]

1 NYC Health + Hospitals/Bellevue, New York, NY, USA

2 Stony Brook University, Stony Brook, NY, USA

*Address all correspondence to: leshya.bokka@stonybrookmedicine.edu

References

[1] Cooley DA. In memoriam: Tribute to René Favaloro, pioneer of coronary bypass. Texas Heart Institute Journal. 2000;**27**(3):231-232

[2] Global Burden of Disease Collaborative Network. Global Burden of Disease Study 2019 (GBD 2019) Results. Seattle, Washington; 2019. p. 2020. Available from: https://vizhub.healthdata.org/gbd-results/

[3] Birger M, Kaldjian AS, Roth GA, Moran AE, Dieleman JL, Bellows BK. Spending on cardiovascular disease and cardiovascular risk factors in the United States: 1996 to 2016. Circulation. 2021;**144**(4):271-282. DOI: 10.1161/circulationaha.120.053216

[4] Healthy People 2030. Heart Disease and Stroke Workgroup. Rockville, MD: Office of Disease Prevention and Health Promotion; 2023. Available from: https://health.gov/healthypeople/about/workgroups/heart-disease-and-stroke-workgroup

[5] Alexander JH, Smith PK. Coronary-artery bypass grafting. The New England Journal of Medicine. 2016;**375**(10):e22

[6] Melly L et al. Fifty years of coronary artery bypass grafting. Journal of Thoracic Disease. 2018;**10**(3):1960-1967

[7] Serruys PW et al. Percutaneous coronary intervention versus coronary-artery bypass grafting for severe coronary artery disease. New England Journal of Medicine. 2009;**360**(10):961-972

[8] Bouabdallaoui N et al. Society of Thoracic Surgeons risk score and EuroSCORE-2 appropriately assess 30-day postoperative mortality in the STICH trial and a contemporary cohort of patients with left ventricular dysfunction undergoing surgical revascularization. Circulation: Heart Failure. 2018;**11**(11):e005531

[9] Lawton JS et al. 2021 ACC/AHA/SCAI guideline for coronary artery revascularization: Executive summary: A report of the American College of Cardiology/American Heart Association joint committee on clinical practice guidelines. Circulation. 2022;**145**(3):e4-e17

[10] Neumann FJ et al. 2018 ESC/EACTS Guidelines on myocardial revascularization. European Heart Journal. 2019;**40**(2):87-165

[11] Velazquez EJ et al. Coronary-artery bypass surgery in patients with ischemic cardiomyopathy. The New England Journal of Medicine. 2016;**374**(16):1511-1520

[12] Maron DJ et al. Initial invasive or conservative strategy for stable coronary disease. The New England Journal of Medicine. 2020;**382**(15):1395-1407

[13] Tatoulis J, Buxton BF, Fuller JA. Patencies of 2127 arterial to coronary conduits over 15 years. The Annals of Thoracic Surgery. 2004;**77**(1):93-101

[14] Sabik JF 3rd et al. Comparison of saphenous vein and internal thoracic artery graft patency by coronary system. The Annals of Thoracic Surgery. 2005;**79**(2):544-551, discussion 544-551

[15] Fitzgibbon GM et al. Coronary bypass graft fate and patient outcome: Angiographic follow-up of 5,065 grafts related to survival and reoperation in 1,388 patients during 25 years. Journal

of the American College of Cardiology. 1996;**28**(3):616-626

[16] Goldman S et al. Long-term patency of saphenous vein and left internal mammary artery grafts after coronary artery bypass surgery: Results from a Department of Veterans Affairs Cooperative Study. Journal of the American College of Cardiology. 2004;**44**(11):2149-2156

[17] Ridderstolpe L et al. Superficial and deep sternal wound complications: Incidence, risk factors and mortality. European Journal of Cardio-Thoracic Surgery. 2001;**20**(6):1168-1175

[18] Taeger CD et al. Changes in sternal perfusion following internal mammary artery bypass surgery. Clinical Hemorheology and Microcirculation. 2017;**67**(1):35-43

[19] Mamchur S, Vecherskii Y, Chichkova T. Influence of internal thoracic artery harvesting on sternal osteoblastic activity and perfusion. Diagnostics (Basel). 2020;**10**(11)

[20] Matsuyama K et al. Sternal closure by rigid plate fixation in off-pump coronary artery bypass grafting: A comparative study. Journal of Artificial Organs. 2016;**19**(2):175-178

[21] Tewarie LS et al. Prevention of sternal dehiscence with the sternum external fixation (stern-E-fix) corset—Randomized trial in 750 patients. Journal of Cardiothoracic Surgery. 2012;7:85

[22] Tomic V et al. Transcriptomic and proteomic patterns of systemic inflammation in on-pump and off-pump coronary artery bypass grafting. Circulation. 2005;**112**(19):2912-2920

[23] Reents W et al. Influence of different autotransfusion devices on the quality of salvaged blood. The Annals of Thoracic Surgery. 1999;**68**(1):58-62

[24] Aldea GS et al. Limitation of thrombin generation, platelet activation, and inflammation by elimination of cardiotomy suction in patients undergoing coronary artery bypass grafting treated with heparin-bonded circuits. The Journal of Thoracic and Cardiovascular Surgery. 2002;**123**(4):742-755

[25] Katz ES et al. Protruding aortic atheromas predict stroke in elderly patients undergoing cardiopulmonary bypass: Experience with intraoperative transesophageal echocardiography. Journal of the American College of Cardiology. 1992;**20**(1):70-77

[26] Gardner TJ et al. Stroke following coronary artery bypass grafting: A ten-year study. The Annals of Thoracic Surgery. 1985;**40**(6):574-581

[27] Balkhy HH et al. Integrating coronary anastomotic connectors and robotics toward a totally endoscopic beating heart approach: Review of 120 cases. The Annals of Thoracic Surgery. 2011;**92**(3):821-827

[28] Balkhy HH et al. Right internal mammary artery use in 140 robotic totally endoscopic coronary bypass cases: Toward multiarterial grafting. Innovations. 2017;**12**(1):9-14

[29] Matschke KE et al. The Cardica C-port system: Clinical and angiographic evaluation of a new device for automated, compliant distal anastomoses in coronary artery bypass grafting surgery—A multicenter prospective clinical trial. The Journal of Thoracic and Cardiovascular Surgery. 2005;**130**(6):1645-1652

[30] Balkhy HH et al. Robotic multivessel endoscopic coronary bypass: Impact of a

beating-heart approach with connectors. The Annals of Thoracic Surgery. 2019;**108**(1):67-73

[31] Hashimoto M, Wehman B, Balkhy HH. Robotic totally endoscopic coronary artery bypass: Tips and tricks for using an anastomotic device. The Journal of Thoracic and Cardiovascular Surgery. 2020;**159**(1):e57-e60

[32] Shapira OM, Mahajna A, Aviel G. Commentary: Automatic distal anastomotic connector—Carrying away a small stone toward moving the entire robotic coronary artery bypass grafting mountain. The Journal of Thoracic and Cardiovascular Surgery. 2020;**159**(1):e61-e62

[33] Göbölös L et al. Robotic totally endoscopic coronary artery bypass grafting: Systematic review of clinical outcomes from the past two decades. Innovations. 2019;**14**(1):5-16

[34] Bonatti J et al. Minimally invasive and robotic coronary artery bypass grafting-a 25-year review. Journal of Thoracic Disease. 2021;**13**(3):1922-1944

[35] Zhao DX et al. Routine intraoperative completion angiography after coronary artery bypass grafting and 1-stop hybrid revascularization results from a fully integrated hybrid catheterization laboratory/operating room. Journal of the American College of Cardiology. 2009;**53**(3):232-241

[36] Puskas JD et al. Hybrid coronary revascularization for the treatment of multivessel coronary artery disease: A Multicenter observational study. Journal of the American College of Cardiology. 2016;**68**(4):356-365

[37] Park SJ et al. Trial of everolimus-eluting stents or bypass surgery for coronary disease. The New England Journal of Medicine. 2015;**372**(13):1204-1212

[38] Peduzzi P, Kamina A, Detre K. Twenty-two-year follow-up in the VA cooperative study of coronary artery bypass surgery for stable angina. The American Journal of Cardiology. 1998;**81**(12):1393-1399

[39] Petrie MC et al. Ten-year outcomes after coronary artery bypass grafting according to age in patients with heart failure and left ventricular systolic dysfunction: An analysis of the extended follow-up of the STICH trial (surgical treatment for ischemic heart failure). Circulation. 2016;**134**(18):1314-1324

[40] Impella5.5® with smart assist®. Instructions for Use & Clinical Reference Manual. Massachusetts: Abiomed; 2024. Available from: https://d1edr79mp9g5zc.cloudfront.net/5eb0affe-1991-449b-bfc0-a5a0516548bf/f4fc23f9-06ae-4e85-9be8-f9e6c72f3f0a/f4fc23f9-06ae-4e85-9be8-f9e6c72f3f0a_viewable_rendition__v.pdf

[41] O'Neill WW et al. A prospective, randomized clinical trial of hemodynamic support with Impella 2.5 versus intra-aortic balloon pump in patients undergoing high-risk percutaneous coronary intervention: The PROTECT II study. Circulation. 2012;**126**(14):1717-1727

[42] Keon WJ et al. Long-term follow-up of coronary endarterectomy. Advances in Cardiology. 1988;**36**:19-26

[43] Livesay JJ et al. Early and late results of coronary endarterectomy. Analysis of 3,369 patients. The Journal of Thoracic and Cardiovascular Surgery. 1986;**92**(4):649-660

[44] Shehada SE et al. Long-term outcomes of coronary endarterectomy in patients with complete imaging follow-up. Seminars in Thoracic

and Cardiovascular Surgery. 2020;**32**(4):730-737

[45] Gill IS et al. Left anterior descending endarterectomy and internal thoracic artery bypass for diffuse coronary disease. The Annals of Thoracic Surgery. 1998;**65**(3):659-662

[46] Brenowitz JB, Kayser KL, Johnson WD. Results of coronary artery endarterectomy and reconstruction. The Journal of Thoracic and Cardiovascular Surgery. 1988;**95**(1):1-10

[47] Goldstein J et al. Angiographic assessment of graft patency after coronary endarterectomy. The Journal of Thoracic and Cardiovascular Surgery. 1991;**102**(4):539-544, discussion 544-545

[48] Frazier OH, March RJ, Horvath KA. Transmyocardial revascularization with a carbon dioxide laser in patients with end-stage coronary artery disease. The New England Journal of Medicine. 1999;**341**(14):1021-1028

[49] Allen KB et al. Comparison of transmyocardial revascularization with medical therapy in patients with refractory angina. The New England Journal of Medicine. 1999;**341**(14):1029-1036

[50] Burkhoff D et al. Transmyocardial laser revascularisation compared with continued medical therapy for treatment of refractory angina pectoris: A prospective randomised trial. ATLANTIC investigators. Angina treatments-lasers and Normal therapies in comparison. Lancet. 1999;**354**(9182):885-890

[51] Jones JW et al. Holmium: YAG laser transmyocardial revascularization relieves angina and improves functional status. The Annals of Thoracic Surgery. 1999;**67**(6):1596-1601, discussion 1601-1602

[52] Allen KB et al. Transmyocardial revascularization: 5-year follow-up of a prospective, randomized multicenter trial. The Annals of Thoracic Surgery. 2004;**77**(4):1228-1234

[53] Horvath KA. Results of prospective randomized controlled trials of transmyocardial laser revascularization. The Heart Surgery Forum. 2002;**5**(1):33-39

[54] Hattler BG et al. Transmyocardial laser revascularization in the patient with unmanageable unstable angina. The Annals of Thoracic Surgery. 1999;**68**(4):1203-1209

[55] Horvath KA et al. Sustained angina relief 5 years after transmyocardial laser revascularization with a CO(2) laser. Circulation. 2001;**104**(12 Suppl. 1):I81-I184

[56] Wehberg KE et al. Improved patient outcomes when transmyocardial revascularization is used as adjunctive revascularization. The Heart Surgery Forum. 2003;**6**(5):328-330

[57] Jones RH et al. Coronary bypass surgery with or without surgical ventricular reconstruction. New England Journal of Medicine. 2009;**360**(17):1705-1717

[58] Investigators; B.A.R.I.B. Comparison of coronary bypass surgery with angioplasty in patients with multivessel disease. The New England Journal of Medicine. 1996;**335**(4):217-225

[59] Flaherty JD, Davidson CJ. Diabetes and coronary revascularization. JAMA. 2005;**293**(12):1501-1508

[60] Farkouh ME et al. Long-term survival following multivessel revascularization in patients with diabetes. Journal of the American College of Cardiology. 2019;**73**(6):629-638

[61] Kappetein AP et al. Treatment of complex coronary artery disease in patients with diabetes: 5-year results comparing outcomes of bypass surgery and percutaneous coronary intervention in the SYNTAX trial. European Journal of Cardio-Thoracic Surgery. 2013;**43**(5):1006-1013

[62] The BARI. 2D study group, a randomized trial of therapies for type 2 diabetes and coronary artery disease. New England Journal of Medicine. 2009;**360**(24):2503-2515

[63] Kugelmass AD et al. The influence of diabetes mellitus on the practice and outcomes of percutaneous coronary intervention in the community: A report from the HCA database. The Journal of Invasive Cardiology. 2003;**15**(10):568-574

[64] Carson JL et al. Diabetes mellitus increases short-term mortality and morbidity in patients undergoing coronary artery bypass graft surgery. Journal of the American College of Cardiology. 2002;**40**(3):418-423

[65] Rabenstein AP et al. Cardiac surgical simulation program during general surgery residency increases resident physician exposure to cardiac surgery and technical expertise. JTCVS Open. 2022;**9**:179-184

Chapter 6

Clinical Follow-Up of Patients after Coronary Artery Bypass Grafting

José Oliveira

Abstract

The follow-up of patients after coronary artery bypass grafting is of paramount importance for a good control of chronic ischemic coronary disease. The non-pharmacological treatment should be approached in an assertive way with the patients, placing it at the center of the problem participating in the health process and definitely understanding the disease. Pharmacological clinical treatment involves modern drugs, widely studied, tested and available worldwide, which need to be used at the maximum tolerated dose in order to achieve the goals disseminated by the guidelines with a view to improving morbidity and mortality and quality of life of patients.

Keywords: by-pass, follow-up, treatment, goals, morbity, mortality

1. Introduction

Coronary heart disease is one of the main causes of mortality worldwide, and coronary artery bypass grafting is one of the forms of treatment for the disease. However, after coronary bypass surgery, the follow-up of patients is of great importance because coronary disease does not cease to exist with surgery and patients continue to fall ill in a natural process of disease evolution, the cardiovascular continuum. Such clinical follow-up should be done strictly with non-pharmacological and pharmacological measures aimed at improving the mortality of patients with chronic coronary heart disease and the morbidity involved, trying to offer the best possible quality of life. The attending cardiologist has the task of always seeking an approximation of the patient with the health-disease process, placing as the main actor of the process to actively participate in the treatment and use the best tools and therapeutic possibilities for each patient to achieve the goals guided by the guidelines.

2. Discussion

IHD (Ischemic Coronary Disease) is one of the major causes of mortality worldwide [1] and its incidence and prevalence have been increasing progressively in much of the globe [2]. This increase has occurred due to the continuous worsening of the lifestyle that we have seen adopted over the last few years by humanity, by which in the final analysis end up increasing the risks of diabetes, arterial hypertension,

IntechOpen

dyslipidemia and obesity [3], considered the great villains of IHD [4]. And an alarming finding is that this has occurred despite great efforts by various agencies around the world with campaigns of primary prevention measures and public initiatives trying to encourage lifestyle changes [5]. Even more worrisome is the fact that there has been a significant increase in young patients affected by the disease [6].

Knowledge about risk factors has improved among people and the understanding of the relationship with cardiovascular disease has also improved [1], however, it is still perceived that there is a long way to go in order to achieve a considerable significant reduction in atherosclerotic disease involvement. Guidelines from around the world recommend lifestyle changes (physical exercise, diets and smoking cessation) and control of risk factors (hypertension, diabetes and dyslipidemia) in addition to drug treatment to minimize the effects of atherosclerosis primarily, but also as a form of secondary prevention combined with some myocardial revascularization therapies in some cases for conorariopathic patients [7]. However, even when this is routinely adopted, there is still a considerable residual risk of major cardiovascular events (MACE): myocardial infarction (MI), stroke, or cardiovascular mortality (CM) [8].

IHD is a disease with typically chronic evolution, with inexorable progression over the years or decades, regardless of any type of treatment that is used [9], that is, although more modern therapies have increased the survival of patients with coronary artery disease, a significant number of them will develop Chronic Coronary Heart Disease (CCHD) at some point in the follow-up [10]. This is because the risk factors continue to overload the myocardial muscle by inflammatory oxidative stress consequent to age, diabetes, hypertension, hypercholesterolemia, sedentary lifestyle, smoking, among others, so it is present both in the genesis of atherosclerosis, as well as in the etiology of IHD and in the progression of CCHD [11]. Annually, 1 in 30 patients with IHD ends up dying due to complications related to the disease, either by Myocardial Infarction (MI), by decompensation of Heart Failure (HF) and/or by arrhythmias consequent to these conditions [12, 13], and about 5–10% of cardiac patients have some cardiovascular event per year [14]. Therefore, reducing the morbidity and mortality involved in CCHD should be our first target in the treatment of patients with this disease [15], as a form of secondary prevention, and to achieve these goals, the treatment of CCHD should be instituted in a rapid, global and rigid manner in all patients [16].

Another factor that justifies the need for assertive treatment of the disease is its important economic impact, since the need for hospital admissions, diagnostic and therapeutic procedures, medical follow-up and continued pharmacological treatment determine a significant economic impact, according to government sources [17]. In the United States, for example, the estimated annual hospital cost for the treatment of events related to ischemic heart disease was US$ 15,540,00 for non-fatal infarction, US$ 2569,00 for stable angina, and US$ 12,058,00 for unstable angina in 1998 [18], and those numbers have been increasing year after year. In Europe, the scenario is the same: in Portugal the DCCC consumed just under 2 billion euros in 2016, equivalent to 1% of that country's GDP (Gross Domestic Product) or 11% of health expenditure at the time [19]; in Belgium in 2004 the estimated cost of the disease was more than 2 billion euros, equivalent to 4000 euros per patient that year [20].

The basis of the treatment of CCHD is the clinical medication [21], instituted years and years ago and increasingly necessary, as confirmed by the largest scientific studies available to date, with the insertion of new drugs more potent, with better results day after day, with lower incidence of undesirable effects and greater symptomatic control of patients [22]. This time, the drug therapy of CCHD has been composed of drugs that slow the progression of the disease, reduce cardiovascular events, improve symptoms and, consequently, quality of life, a fact elucidated by evidence on the reduction of angina cases [23]. This has contributed to not further worsen mortality and promote better quality of life among patients [24], since the treatment instituted prevents ventricular remodeling, preserves the myocardium and ventricular function, reduces sudden death and improves the functional class and prognosis of the sick [25].

Allied to the optimized drug treatment, the various modes of secondary prevention are already well known, as we have said, such as lifestyle changes (abandonment of sedentary lifestyle, adherence to diets known to be cardioprotective, combating obesity and smoking cessation, mainly) [26] and combating modifiable risk factors such as hypertension, diabetes and hypercholesterolemia, especially [27]. However, on the one hand, we have still noticed a very persevering therapeutic inertia among cardiologist medical professionals with little prescription of what is considered the best possible treatment [28] and on the other, little adherence on the part of patients to what has been prescribed [29]. This is an unacceptable reality since it is recognized that good adherence to optimized cardiac therapies could be associated with a 35% reduction in mortality risk from any cause in patients with CHD [30].

On the part of physicians, such inertia is erroneously justified, in part because they accept that patients being asymptomatic, for example in the postoperative period of coronary artery bypass graft surgery, are well treated, but do not pay attention to the so-called therapeutic targets already widely disseminated by international Guidelines. On the part of patients, the lack of adherence to the proposed treatment often finds justification because they do not truly know the problem they have, because often the doctors who treat it do not express themselves convincingly, they cannot make patients understand how important the subsequent treatment is. To reverse the situation, it is up to cardiologists to apply the best available evidence, which is constantly updated and widely disseminated around the world and a good persuasion training with patients and families to understand the dimension of the problem and the real benefit of the proposed treatments.

Part of the non-pharmacological treatment known to be beneficial in CCHD is the abandonment of sedentary lifestyle and stimulation of physical exercises. In fact, it has long been known that it is important that such practices are important to improve cardiovascular health in the postoperative period of Coronary Artery Bypass Graft surgery (CABG), with several studies demonstrating that patients with CCHD, who participate in regular physical training programs, and who receive guidance on the control of risk factors for cardiovascular diseases, have a lower number of postoperative events and hospital readmissions and reduced mortality [31]. However, very little is addressed in a real and practical way these orientations and the patients even understand that this conduct is really necessary, but they are not really oriented to adopt it as a daily practice or in a correct, continuous way. Thus, stimulating the practice of daily physical activities, preferably in cardiac rehabilitation programs, reduces cardiac and all-cause mortality [32].

Likewise, it is well known of all the harms of tobacco for heart health, and patients who maintain addiction after CABG surgery have a higher chance of death than those patients who do not [33]. However, it is estimated that although 70% of smokers wish at some point to stop the addiction, only 1/3 of them can actually do so [34]. This is because many of them simply do not understand the reasons why they should quit smoking or do not feel encouraged to take action since they do not have precise guidance on the risks and problems involved with addiction. It is up to the cardiologist to openly address the topic, explaining the real harms, the ways in which tobacco degrades the circulatory system and heart, but also addressing benefits that are obtained by quitting tobacco and how to proceed to achieve success in quitting smoking. Several techniques of psychotherapy or daily habits associated or not pharmacological treatments have been employed in several parts with expressive results [35]. It is essential to identify situations and strategies that can improve the effectiveness of treatments for tobacco use and in all therapeutic approaches, smoking cessation is one of the most crucial factors [36].

Another very important factor in the non-drug treatment of CCHD is diet, since it is known that diet has a key role in the progression of ischemic heart disease, since the intake of diets rich in saturated fat, calories and salt can result in greater lack of control of the main risk factors for CHCD: obesity, hypertension, diabetes and hypercholesterolemia [37]. Thus, the re-education of dietary habits represents an important intervention in the secondary prevention of ischemic heart disease and its indication is based on several clinical evidences [38]. Epidemiological, observational and intervention studies have demonstrated the positive influence of a balanced diet on the primary and secondary prevention of cardiovascular events in the postoperative period of CABG and in the follow-up of the CCHCD and dietary patterns free of trans fats reduced in saturated fats, sugars, rich in fiber, unsaturated fats and complex carbohydrates demonstrate an inverse association with the development of cardiovascular disease, presenting positive action in the control of metabolic disorders [39]. Likewise, the harmful effects of alcohol on the cardiovascular system of patients with CHCD are widely known [40], so that the consumption of alcoholic beverages should be discouraged in all patients.

In addition to these so-called conventional risk factors, some others have been cited as adjuvants in CCHD, including environmental pollution [41], stress [42], respiratory infections [43], among others, which also need to be prevented and treated. Finally, some morbidities should also be investigated and addressed, under penalty of compromising the good evolution of patients with CHCD, such as: hypothyroidism [44], chronic kidney disease [45], atrial fibrillation [46], among others.

When it comes to clinical drug treatment, as we have commented, a considerable range of drugs has been tested and approved for what is called Optimized Drug Treatment, which should be widely instituted in all patients with CHD, unless there is some important contraindication or undesirable effect limiting the use. The basis of BMT encompasses the use of prognostic-modifying and cardioprotective medications such as angiotensin-converting enzyme inhibitors or angiotensin receptor blockers, beta-blockers (and other sinus node blockers), statins, and antiplatelet agents for all patients [25], in addition to mineracolocorticoid inhibitors in some specific situations, as well as sodium-glucose co-transporter inhibitors (SGLT2) and symptomatic medications such as nitrates and other vasodilators, diuretics, among others, as we will discuss below. Such treatment should be employed to avoid undesirable outcomes such as death, myocardial infarction and/or heart failure (HF), which is the final pathway of cardiac diseases, invariably. However, when HF is developed, other strategies are employed to reduce mortality and prevent sudden death, improve symptoms and readmissions and the prognosis of patients, such as the use of implantable cardiodefibrillator (ICD) or resynchronizer, and heart transplantation in specific cases [47].

Specifically in relation to antiplatelet agents, acetylsalicylic acid (ASA) is the first choice because it reduces, on average, by 33% the risk of cardiovascular events in patients with CCHD [48], should always be prescribed in all patients, except for rare cases of contraindication (allergy or intolerance, active bleeding, hemophilia and active peptic ulcer) or high probability of gastrointestinal or genitourinary bleeding, with degree of recommendation I, level of evidence A [49], at a dose of 75–325 mg/day [50]. Other platelet antiaggregants such as P2Y12 enzyme inhibitors (clopidogrel, prasugrel and ticagrelor) play a key role in increasing the prevention of coronary thrombogenesis, being used in association with ASA or in substitution for it when there is an absolute contraindication to its use [49], with excellent results. The Clopidogrel vs. Aspirin in Patients at Risk of Ischaemic Events (CAPRIE) study showed a slight overall benefit of clopidogrel use over ASA with a better safety profile in preventing undesirable cardiovascular outcomes [51], should be used at a dose of 75 mg/day in association with aspirin (ASA) if there is MI for 1 year and ad eternum if there is a high risk of new coronary events, and this period may be reduced depending on careful individual evaluation taking into account bleeding risk and benefit of extended antiplatelet aggregation [52]. Prasugrel, on the other hand, has a faster, more predictable onset of action and, on average, a greater antiplatelet effect than clopidogrel, with greater efficacy in aspirin patients undergoing percutaneous coronary intervention (PCI), but not in patients only clinically treated [53], however, on the other hand, it has a higher risk of bleeding and should be used with caution in patients with a history of stroke, older than 70 years and less than 60 kg of body weight [54]. Finally, Ticagrelor has a more predictable and consistent higher level of P2Y12 inhibition during maintenance treatment of patients adhering to treatment [55], and also faster onset of action than clopidogrel [56], in addition to similar efficacy and safety to aspirin when monotherapy [57], at a dose of 90 mg 2 x daily, however, more prone to bleeding [58].

Incidentally in specific cases is indicated the double antiplatelet aggregation terapy (DAPT), being always necessary the presence of aspirin associated with one of the P2Y12 inhibitors mentioned, such as: in general, infarcted patients who are submitted to CABG should receive DAPT for 1 year or in those with CCHD who were affected by AMI, as well as in those post-CABG in which a subsequent percutaneous coronary intervention (PCI) was required who should receive DAPT for at least 6 months to 1 year, depending on the type of coronary stent used and/or the benefit of maintaining therapy versus risk of bleeding, digestive, or other fatal and non-fatal [59]. In order to protect the patient from gastric bleeding, a proton pump inhibitor (PPI) such as pantoprazole at a dose of 40 mg/day for example (but not omeprazole or esomeprazole) can be used, since they reduce the risk of gastrointestinal bleeding in patients treated with DAPT and can be used with some safety [60].

In relation to other anti-thrombotic drugs, anticoagulants are currently accurately indicated if there is a rhythm of Atrial Fibrillation (AF) at any time, replacing all the antiaggregants mentioned above, and therapy is recommended in patients with CCHD and such arrhythmia to reduce the risk of ischemic events, especially cerebral, since they have been shown to be superior in this prevention in relation to monotherapy with aspirin or another P2Y12 inhibitor or DAPT [61]. On the other hand, in sinus rhythm, antiplatelet therapy associated with the use of anticoagulants, even at low doses to prevent new ischemic events, is still controversial and lacks further evidence [62].

Post-CABG dyslipidemia should be managed rigorously, following therapeutic targets already defined by guidelines based on pharmacological treatment and lifestyle change [63]. Such patients are considered to be at very high cardiovascular risk and therefore should have LDL-cholesterol reduced to less than 50 mg/dL or even lower in order to avoid further ischemic events [7]. The basis of pharmacological treatment is with statins at the maximum possible and well-tolerated dose (rosuvastatin

40 mg/day or atorvastatin 80 mg/day) and, when target LDL-cholesterol levels are not reached with statins alone, the combination of ezetimibe at a dose of 10 mg/day is indicated [64]. In recent years new antilipemics have been included in the list of treatment of dyslipidemias and in this scenario fit the molecules inhibitory of the conversion of the liver enzyme in the active metabolite PCSK9 (evolocumab and alirocumab), which guarantee an even greater reduction of LDL levels, and should be used when reaching the maximum dose of statins in association with ezetimibe and has not yet reached the recommended target level [15]. Such drugs, in robust trials, have demonstrated a great potential to reduce LDL-cholesterol levels, with interesting ischemic protection and with an equally encouraging safety and tolerability profile, being used in subcutaneous applications every 15 days. More recently, inclisiran, an inhibitor of hepatic synthesis of the enzyme PCSK9 whose LDL-cholesterol-lowering effect has been sustained in clinical studies with subcutaneous applications every 6 months, and an acceptable safety profile [65].

In addition to those already mentioned, an equally important pharmacological class for the treatment of patients after CABG and which, as we have said, is part of the basic therapeutic arsenal of these patients, are the Angiotensin-Converting Enzyme (ACEi) Inhibitors, whose main representatives are: enalapril up to 40 mg/day, captopril up to 150 mg/day, ramipril up to 10 mg/day plus lisinopril and peridonpril. They have been shown to be beneficial in the prevention of death, AMI and stroke and have an important role in minimizing the occurrence of ischemic events after CABG, and should be administered early to all patients with ventricular dysfunction, due to the advantages of these drugs in relation to cardiac remodeling and hemodynamic improvement (vasodilation and reduction of afterload) generating a decrease in mortality and acting as anti-ischemics, through its protective effects of the vascular bed (antiatherosclerotic, antithrombotic and anti-inflammatory) [66]. A not infrequent side effect of ACEi is dry cough, which can be an impediment to continuous use, and in these cases should be replaced by Angiotensin II Receptor Blockers (ARBs), whose most used representatives are: losartan up to 100 mg/day, valsartan up to 320 mg/day, candesartan up to 32 mg/day, olmesartan up to 40 mg/day. ARBs seem to be as effective as, or possibly slightly less effective than, ACEi when compared directly [67], and, therefore, although the reduction in mortality and hospitalization has been demonstrated with these drugs in some studies with patients intolerant to ACEi, due to the greater number of evidences, ACE inhibitors remain the medication of choice, ARBs being a reasonable alternative [68]. ACEi or ARBs are indicated up to the maximum tolerated dose in order to obtain maximum SBP (systolic blood pressure) below 130 mmHg and DBP (diastolic blood pressure) below 90 mmHg, and when such values are not obtained, the association with thiazide diuretics such as hydrochlorothiazide at the maximum dose of 50 mg/day should be considered, Other options being dihydropyridine calcium channel blockers as amlodipine up to 10 mg/day, levanlodipine up to 5 mg/day, nifedipine up to 60 mg/day or nitrendpine, lercanidipine, felodipine [69].

More recent studies have identified neprilysin, an endogenous enzyme that degrades vasoactive peptides such as bradycin and natriuretic peptides and the inhibition of this enzyme by the sacubitril-valsartan combination has shown very satisfactory results generating diuretic and natriuretic effect, myocardial relaxation anti-remodeling and reduction of renin-aldoesterone, known vasoconstrictors. Its use has been recommended in patients after CABG, especially in patients with dyspnea, in efforts to reduce cases of re-hospitalization for heart failure (HF) and death [70].

Beta-blockers (metoprolol up to 200 mg/day, atenolol up to 100 mg/day, carvedilol up to 100 mg/day, nebivolol up to 10 mg/day or bisoprolol up to 10 mg/day) also make up the basic treatment for post-CABG patients, since patients must maintain heart rate (HR) between 55 and 60 BPM at rest sinus rhythm [71], in order to ensure the best benefit, which is an important reduction in mortality and/or cardiovascular events [72]. If such a HR index cannot be achieved, the association with non-dihydropyridine calcium channel blockers (verapamil up to 480 mg/day or diltiazem up to 240 mg/day) may be necessary, although its increase in clinical benefit is uncertain and has potential undesirable effects such as bradyarrhythmias and/or atrioventricular blocks [73]. Another option to be associated with non-dihydropyridine beta-blockers and/or BCCs in the control of HR is ivabradine (at a maximum dose of 15 mg/day), which has shown good results in increasing exercise tolerance, increasing the effort-induced ischemic threshold and reducing effort-induced angina [74].

As we have already mentioned, aldosterone blockade is an important pharmacological treatment route of CCHD, especially in those patients who develop HF and/or reduced ejection fraction (EF) on echocardiogram, and this is also possible with mineralocorticoid inhibitors such as spironolactone (25–50 mg/day) and eplerenone (25–50 mg/day). The use of such medications was associated with lower mortality and hospitalization rates, as well as lower vascular and myocardial fibrosis in this type of patient [75], eplerenone, being a more selective inhibitor, has a more pronounced effect and less side effect of gynecomastia and erectile sexual dysfunction than spironolactone [76]. Similarly, patients with CCHD after CABG who develop some degree of HF should receive SGLT2 inhibitors (empaglifozine up to 25 mg/day and dapaglifozine up to 10 mg/day), which inhibit glucose reabsorption in the proximal convoluted tubule, resulting in glycosuria and reduced glycemic levels [77] and improve left ventricular parietal tension secondary to decreased pre- (effect of natriuresis and osmotic diuresis) and afterload (improvement in endothelial function and reduced blood pressure) [78], improve cardiomyocyte metabolism and bioenergetics (increased ketogenesis and increased β-hydroxybutyrate supply), inhibit the myocardial sodium-hydrogen pump (which leads to higher calcium concentration in the mitochondria), reduce cardiac necrosis and fibrosis (inhibition of collagen synthesis), and decrease cytokine production in epicardial fatty tissue [79]. Such effects guarantee in these patients a significant reduction in the main adverse cardiovascular events: cardiovascular death, AMI and stroke, and a surprising reduction in hospitalization for heart failure [80], in addition to improved quality of life and renal protection [81].

In patients who still remain symptomatic for angina after CABG, it is crucial to identify if there is no *de novo* obstructive coronary disease by means of follow-up exams such as cineangiochonariography and/or myocardial scintigraphy/echostress for example and once the presence of arterial obstruction is excluded, improve the antianginal treatment, which can be done with short-acting nitrates (such as isosorbide dinitrate 5 mg) or long-acting (such as isosorbide mononitrate up to 60 mg) mg/day, and other medications, which have adjuvant power and should be used when the patient is on the maximum tolerated dose of beta-blockers [7]. Trimetazidine (35 mg 12/12 h or 80 mg single daily dose) is an antianginal with neutral hemodynamic effect that in addition to beta-blocker improves effort-induced myocardial ischemia more than other antianginal drugs [82], which supports the indication of its use as a second line of medications in patients with BMT and still persistently anginal [7]. Other available options of anti-anginal drugs such as nicorandil and ranolazine are also possible but with fewer indications for the treatment of patients with CCHD and have use considered an exception by the largest studies carried out, since although they reasonably improve angina have possible undesirable effects that discourage the use such as nausea, increased QT interval, gastrointestinal ulcerations, constipation, among others [7], moreover, the studies revealed that such medications did not interfere, in a statistically justifiable way, in the reduction of the compound of hard events (AMI, cardiac death and stroke) [83].

It is perceived that the range of treatment for CCHD is immense, however, a major obstacle, as has been said, to achieve goals and the maximum benefit that the treatment can offer is adherence to treatment by patients. Studies have emphasized that low adherence to treatment, both pharmacological and non-pharmacological, is among the main destabilizing factors of CCHD [84] and because of this, readmission rates remain high [85]. Several studies have shown that low adherence to treatment would be related to risk factors involving socioeconomic problems, psychological disorders and cognitive impairments, added to the characteristics of the disease and the complexity of the treatment. In addition, the costs of medications, the quantities and their effects, the relationship between health professional and patient and the various types of support given are factors that contribute to influence treatment adherence [86]. Alarming numbers, such as 50% adherence to optimized pharmacological treatment and only 20% adherence to non-pharmacological guidelines, have been found in studies with CCHD [86], a frightening scenario that needs to be urgently reversed with systematic education of patients and more frequent follow-up by attending physicians, in search of the best for each patient.

Special attention deserves some questions and doubts brought by patients in relation to some factors in the post-CABG such as hormone replacement for example, use of medications for erectile dysfunction and testosterone replacement, consent to sexual activities, vitamin replacement and vaccination in general.

Regarding hormone replacement, some controversies are old, but the current trend is towards non-indication for cardiovascular protection, since the results of large randomized studies have shown that replacement does not improve cardiac prognosis and increases the risk of more severe cardiovascular disease in women after 60 years of age [7]. In addition, smokers and obese women should be encouraged to lose weight and stop the addiction and if it is not possible, hormone replacement is even more preventive, despite greatly increasing the risk of thromboembolic phenomena.

In the case of erectile dysfunction it is known that such a condition is an important predictor for more serious cardiovascular diseases in post-CABG patients and a high percentage of patients after CABG have some erectile disorder. Even the association with coronary artery disease is the cause of erectile dysfunction, in general, especially if the patient is diabetic, and not the use of medications (such as beta-blockers, ACE inhibitors, statins, etc.) to treat CHCD as is thought, although the evidence is limited and conflicting. Usually if erectile symptoms occurred within 4 weeks of starting treatment for CCHD the cause may actually be medications and other therapeutic options may be tried, but if they occur after 4 weeks of use, other causes should be investigated. On the other hand, drug therapies for erectile dysfunction do not increase the cardiovascular risk in patients with CHCD after CABG and can be indicated in stable patients, if necessary, as long as they are not using nitrates and do not use doses higher than the maximum recommended as safe, and special attention should be paid to more hypotensive patients [87].

Incidentally a frequent doubt in the follow-up of post-CABG patients is the return to sexual activities. The fear of the occurrence of cardiac complications during sexual intercourse is responsible for most of the changes in sexual dysfunction that occurs in patients with heart disease after CABG, and it is reported that 17% of patients and 35% of their spouses are afraid to resume sexual activities and 39% of patients reduce their practice after having undergone this type of treatment. However since the creation of man sexual activity is part of our day-to-day and it has light metabolic expenditure, because the maximum cardiac effort does not exceed more than 10–15 seconds, reaching maximum heart rate between 90 and 144 bpm, and similar to climbing two flights of stairs, walking hurriedly or performing common tasks in various occupations [88], so that the cardiac patient after CABG, as he feels safe, less symptomatic, and after 3–4 weeks which is the approximate time of bone healing of the sternotomy, you can be released to practice your sexual activities normally.

Testosterone, in turn, as we know, has androgenic and anabolic effects, but also exerts an effect on the vascular bed, promoting vasodilation through the release of nitric oxide and modulation of calcium channels, which impacts endothelial function. In patients with coronary artery disease (CAD) and heart failure (HF), reductions in total testosterone concentrations are related to higher mortality and severity of these diseases, however, although the effects of testosterone on the increase of muscle mass and muscle strength are well established in the literature, the effects of this substance on the cardiovascular system need to be better elucidated [89], studies have shown that exogenous replacement is related to changes in the lipid profile (reduction of HDL and increase in LDL), morphological and functional changes of the left ventricle, hemodynamic changes and autonomic alterations [90], which makes it still not well regarded and controversial for the treatment of patients with CCHD after CABG [87].

Vitamins and supplements have emerged in droves these days with promises of improving cardiac performance. The association between hypovitaminosis and inflammatory markers and subclinical atherosclerosis has been reported in several studies, generally cross-sectional and small and deficiency of some vitamins has been associated with both endothelial dysfunction, reflected by lower brachial artery flow-mediated dilation as to the greater carotid intima-medial thickness in different patient profiles [91]. Still some studies have even shown that the status of vitamin D for example can also influence the prognosis of individuals already affected by AMI and in elderly with stable HF have significantly lower concentrations of 25(OH)D, verifying among these a prevalence of hypovitaminosis D of almost 100% [92]. However, a recent population survey in the United States showed that the prevalence of hypovitaminosis D has been increasing in recent years, currently affecting up to 90.0% of pigmented populations (black, Hispanic and Asian) and around 3/4 of the white population, especially in older patients [93]. Therefore, it is not yet clear whether hypovitaminosis D is an important risk factor for heart disease or occurs at random due to the age of those affected with the disease and data from randomized studies to evaluate the impact of vitamin D supplementation in patients with coronary artery disease after CABG on their cardiovascular risk are limited, especially in relation to hard outcomes, and have sometimes reported conflicting results [92]. As seen, some hypovitaminosis is an emerging public health problem in the world, with important implications for cardiovascular morbidity and mortality, but there is still a lack of sufficient evidence, based on large randomized and placebo-controlled studies, with long-term follow-up and with adequate statistical power to evaluate hard outcomes in patients with coronary artery disease after CABGV and only in this way can the role of vitamin supplementation in the prevention and treatment of these patients be definitively established.

Finally, the need for influenza vaccination in patients with heart disease was determined first by historical reports of increased mortality in epidemics and, later, by epidemiological studies and today, it is known that annual vaccination is an effective measure in secondary prevention, as it reduces hospital admissions for HF, stroke and AMI in post-CABG patients, in addition to reducing overall mortality more significantly than many drugs or interventions [93]. On the other hand, since the first series published from China and Italy, the severity of COVID-19 has stood out in the carriers of chronic non-communicable diseases such as those with CHD after CABG, most likely taken in common by chronic systemic inflammation, so that currently this group of patients must also be vaccinated against COVID, In the light of current knowledge [94], however, it remains to better define the periodicity of vaccination indication or vaccination schedule. In addition, it is known that patients with post-CABG CHCD have an increased chance of presenting decompensation of the disease at some point and hospitalization for HF and, in a nosocomial environment, patients with HF have an increased risk of pulmonary infections, especially pneumonia, thus, vaccination against respiratory infections by pneumococci is also cost-effective as a public health measure [95].

The clinical evolution of coronary patients after CABG tends to be benign, but some cases may present complications in the follow-up, and therefore this should be done often, with routine consultations every 6 months in the first year after surgery, at most, because the chance of developing exacerbations of the disease and the appearance of HF is great due to systolic and/or diastolic dysfunction due to myocardial injury caused by chonaropathy [7]. And it is recognized that there is a risk of more evident complications in symptomatic patients but also in oligo or asymptomatic patients, so that in the consultations an active search for HF symptoms should be made, with special attention to the search for exercise intolerance and dyspnea to exertion in addition to the search for associated angina or equivalent, assessment of adherence to recommended therapy, physical activities and diet [7]. In the clinical examination it is necessary to check the nutritional status and make active research for signs of HF such as leg edema, presence of signs of HF such as jugular stasis, hepatomegaly, sacral edema/anasarca, pulmonary crepitation, among others, and also evaluate heart rate and blood pressure and know how the pressure levels are outside the office environment for therapeutic optimization in addition to cardiac auscultation in order to search for heart murmurs and/or muffling of sounds [7].

In the periodic evaluation of complementary exams, the routine electrocardiogram, which provides information on heart rate and rhythm, as well as possible identification of arrhythmias and conduction disorders and signs of overload of cardiac chambers, and echocardiogram for evaluation of cardiac chambers, systolic and/or diastolic dysfunction, of the ejection fraction, appear as crucial options. The presence of cavitary thrombi and other complications as indirect signs of pulmonary hypertension and valve dysfunction, among others [7]. The chest X-ray, in turn, is useful for identifying signs of pulmonary congestion, interstitial edema and investigation of pleural effusions7 and blood laboratory tests serve for the objective evaluation of nitrogenous slags and subjective renal function, investigation of electrolyte disturbances and evaluation/follow-up/treatment of metabolic diseases such as thyroidopathy, diabetes and hypercholesterolemia in addition to the identification of possible complicating factors such as hyperuricemia, liver diseases, among others [7]. It should be noted, however, that although there is some additional prognostic value in the use of several serological biomarkers (such as BNP, CRP, among others) individually or in association with each other, there is currently no evidence that routine use ensures better evaluation and care [7].

All this evaluation is of paramount importance because post-CABG patients are recognized as having very high cardiovascular risk and as such should have the laboratory and hemodynamic targets sought at all times, in order to minimize the risk of secondary HF, need for new revascularization (percutaneous or surgical), death or other complications, which may be more impactful in the first year after surgery. After 1 year of CABG, annual consultations are sufficient in patients with good evolution and in patients with some complication identified by complementary tests, or in those at high risk for them, or who have symptoms at some point again a more rigorous follow-up is necessary [7].

Other equally important tests for follow-up are the 24-hour holter and 7–20 day lopper, which can help in the search for arrhythmias and/or evaluation of symptoms such as dizziness, palpitation, among others and signs such as syncope or pre-syncope, for example. Similarly, a TILT-test may be indicated in special situations and carotid and lower extremity Doppler if concomitant vascular obstruction at other arterial sites is suspected. In cases where the echocardiogram is not elucidative or if there is the intention to investigate the presence of myocardial fibrosis or infiltrative myocardial diseases, magnetic resonance imaging is highly indicated. If the idea is functional evaluation of the patient with a view to release for physical activity practices and/or research of stress-induced signs/symptoms, the treadmill exercise test is highly indicated.

Finally, in patients with unequivocal persistent symptoms of *de novo* coronary obstruction, such as angina on exertion, for example despite the optimized drug treatment and the recommended therapeutic goals have been achieved, a new evaluation for the investigation of metabolic alterations and myocardial ischemic suffering can be used as scintigraphy or other imaging tests with stress such as echocardiography, for example [96]. If there is indeed ischemia demonstrated by such tests and/or the patient remains symptomatic, a new coronary angiography may be more elucidative and define better forms of treatment.

It is noticed, therefore, that the prognosis of post-CABG patients will depend on a number of factors such as the presence of comorbidities such as diabetes, dyslipidemias, advanced age, obesity, smoking, degree of physical activity and adherence to healthy living practices (diet, etc.) prior to surgery, in addition to the concomitant presence of cancer, arterial obstructions in other arterial sites, hepato or nephropathies or other systemic diseases. It is also recognized that the presence of symptoms of angina and/or dyspnea after CABG or equivalent also mean a worse prognosis of patients with CHCD, as well as arrhythmias on exertion or at rest and especially adherence to the proposed drug therapy. They also have a considerable influence on the anatomical-morphological-functional aspects of the cardiac chambers seen by echocardiogram and/or resonance imaging and the presence of new coronary obstructions after CABG with or without the need for new revascularization.

3. Conclusion

As seen, the post-CABG treatment is extremely important and follow-up of patients of paramount necessity, since the disease has a progressive character and the evolution to hard outcomes seems inexorable. The attending cardiologist takes a broad, rigorous and continuous approach placing the patient in the center of attention with an understanding of the disease, clear and objective explanations. Always attentive to the recommended goals and adopting the best available evidence with the most cost-effective treatment to achieve them and with great empathy with the patient in order to provide improvement in overall mortality, morbidity and quality of life.

Conflict of interest

The author has no conflict of interest.

Author details

José Oliveira
NCOR Clinic, Itajubá, Brazil

*Address all correspondence to: jotamedicina@yahoo.com.br

References

[1] Benjamin EJ, Muntner P, Alonso A, Bittencourt MS, Callaway CW, Carson AP, et al. Heart disease and stroke statistics—2019 update: A report from the American Heart Association. Circulation. 2019;**139**:56-e528

[2] Reza M et al. Cardiovascular disease projections in the United States based on the 2020 census estimates. Journal of the American College of Cardiology. 2022;**80**(6):565-578

[3] Mehta D. Integrative medicine and cardiovascular disorders. Primary Care. 2017;**44**(2):351-367

[4] Wong ND et al. Metabolic syndrome, diabetes, and incidence and progression of coronary calcium. JACC: Cardiovascular Imaging. 2012;**5**:358-366

[5] Roth GA, Forouzanfar MH, Moran AE, Barber R, Nguyen G, Feigin VL, et al. Demographic and epidemiologic drivers of global cardiovascular mortality. The New England Journal of Medicine. 2015;**372**:1333-1341

[6] Arora S et al. Twenty year trends and sex differences in young adults hospitalized with acute myocardial infarction: The ARIC community surveillance study. Circulation. 2019;**139**:1047-1056

[7] Knuuti J et al. ESC scientific document group. 2019 ESC guidelines for the diagnosis and management of chronic coronary syndromes. European Heart Journal. 2020;**41**:407-477

[8] Fiolet ATL et al. Efficacy and safety of low-dose colchicine in patients with coronary disease: A systematic review and meta-analysis of randomized trials. European Heart Journal. 2021;**42**:2765-2775

[9] Soares A et al. Death and myocardial infarction following initial revascularization versus optimal medical therapy in chronic coronary syndromes with myocardial ischemia: A systematic review and meta-analysis of contemporary randomized controlled trials. Journal of the American Heart Association. 2021;**10**:019114

[10] Barbosa JE et al. Perfil da Expressão do mRNA do Nrf2, NF-κB e PPARβ/δ em Pacientes com Doença Arterial Coronariana. Arquivos Brasileiros de Cardiologia. 2019;**113**(6):1121-1127

[11] Ezekowitz JA. Is there a sex gap in surviving an acute coronary syndrome or subsequent development of heart failure? Circulation. 2020;**142**:2231-2239

[12] Fox KAA, Metra M, Morais J, Atar D. The myth of "stable" coronary artery disease. Nature Reviews. Cardiology. 2020;**17**:9-21

[13] Sabatine MS et al. Evolocumab and clinical outcomes in patients with cardiovascular disease. The New England Journal of Medicine. 2017;**376**:1713-1722

[14] Eikelboom JW et al. Rivaroxaban with or without aspirin in stable cardiovascular disease. The New England Journal of Medicine. 2017;**377**:1319-1330

[15] Schwartz GG et al. Alirocumab and cardiovascular outcomes after acute coronary syndrome. The New England Journal of Medicine. 2018;**379**:2097-2107

[16] Maron DJ et al. Initial invasive or conservative strategy for stable coronary

disease. The New England Journal of Medicine. 2020;**382**(15):1395-1407

[17] Ribeiro RA et al. Custo Anual do Manejo da Cardiopatia Isquêmica Crônica no Brasil. Perspectiva Pública e Privada. Arquivos Brasileiros de Cardiologia. 2005;**85**:1-6

[18] Stewart S, Murphy N, Walker A, McGuire A, McMurray JJ. The current cost of angina pectoris to the National Health Service in the UK. Heart. 2003;**89**:848-853

[19] Costa J et al. Atherosclerosis: The cost of illness in Portugal. Revista Portuguesa de Cardiologia. 2021;**40**(6):409-419

[20] Vlayen J, De Backer G, Peers J, et al. Atherosclerotic cardiovascular diseases in Belgium: A cost-of-illness analysis. Cardiovascular Drugs and Therapy. 2008;**22**:487-494

[21] Ramires JF, Jordão MR, Fernandes F, Mady C. Impacto dos novos estudos clínicos no tratamento da insuficiência cardíaca. A Sociedade de Cardiologia do Estado de São Paulo. 2015;**25**(2):90-93

[22] Boden WE, O'Rourke RA, Teo KK, Hartigan PM, Maron DJ, Kostuk WJ, et al. Optimal medical therapy with or without PCI for stable coronary disease. The New England Journal of Medicine. 2007;**356**(15):1503-1516

[23] Padala SK, Lavelle MP, Sidhu MS, Cabral KP, Morrone D, Boden WE, et al. Antianginal therapy for stable ischemic heart disease: A contemporary review. Journal of Cardiovascular Pharmacology and Therapeutics. 2017;**22**:499-510

[24] Simões MV, Schwartzmann PV, Marques F. Sistema peptídeo natriurético em insuficiência cardíaca: perspectivas no diagnóstico e no tratamento. A Sociedade de Cardiologia do Estado de São Paulo. 2015;**25**(2):62-68

[25] Santos EB, Bianco HT. Atualizações em doença cardíaca isquêmica aguda e crônica. Revista da Sociedade Brasileira de Clínica Médica. 2018;**16**(1):52-58

[26] Forman DE, Sanderson BK, Josephson RA, Raikhelkar J, BittnerV. AmericanCollegeofCardiology's prevention of cardiovascular disease section. Heart failure as a newly approved diagnosis for cardiac rehabilitation: challenges and opportunities. Journal of the American College of Cardiology. 2015;**65**:26529

[27] Santa GBA et al. Tendência Temporal da Mortalidade por Doenças Isquêmicas do Coração no Nordeste Brasileiro (1996-2016): Uma Análise Segundo Gênero e Faixa Etária. Arquivos Brasileiros de Cardiologia. 2021;**117**(1):51-60

[28] Xavier HT et al. V Diretriz Brasileira de Dislipidemias e Prevenção da Aterosclerose. Arquivos Brasileiros de Cardiologia. 2013;**101**:1-22

[29] Sobral PD, Gomes ET, Carvalho PO, Godoi ET, Oliveira DC. Prevalência de adesão medicamentosa em pacientes com doença arterial coronariana crônica. Enfermagem Brasil. 2020;**19**(2):98-104

[30] Naderi SH, Bestwick JP, Wald DS. Adherence to drugs that prevent cardiovascular disease: Meta-analysis on 376,162 patients. The American Journal of Medicine. 2012;**125**(9):882-887

[31] Nery RM, Barbisan JN, Mahmud MI. Influência da prática da atividade física no resultado da cirurgia de revascularização miocárdica. Revista Brasileira de Cirurgia Cardiovascular. 2007;**22**(3):297-302

[32] Taylor RS, Brown A, Ebrahim S, Jolliffe J, Noorani H, Rees K, et al. Exercise-based rehabilitation for patients with coronary heart disease: Systematic

review and meta-analysis of randomized controlled trials. The American Journal of Medicine. 2004;**116**(10):682-689

[33] Pietrobom RC, Barbisan JN. Impact of coronary artery bypass graft surgery in smoking cessation. Revista Brasileira de Cirurgia Cardiovascular. 2010;**25**(1):79-84

[34] Rigotti NA. Clinical practice. Treatment of tobacco use and dependence. The New England Journal of Medicine. 2002;**346**(7):506-512

[35] Barth J, Critchley J, Bengel J. Efficacy of psychosocial interventions for smoking cessation in patients with coronary heart disease: A systematic review and meta-analysis. Annals of Behavioral Medicine. 2006;**32**(1):10-20

[36] NIH State-of-the-Science Panel. National Institutes of Health state-of-the-science conference statement: Tobacco use: Prevention, cessation, and control. Annals of Internal Medicine. 2006;**145**(11):839-844

[37] Lakka TA, Bouchard C. Physical activity, obesity and cardiovascular diseases. Handbook of Experimental Pharmacology. 2005;**170**:137-163

[38] Pinheiro DGM, Pinheiro CHJ, Marinho MJF. Lifestyle and the importance of health education in the cardiac rehabilitation after myocardial revascularization surgery. Revista Brasileira em Promoção da Saúde. 2007;**20**(4):213-220

[39] Ferreira GAI et al. Analysis of dietary intake and nutritional status of subjects submitted to elective cardiac surgery at a public reference hospital in cardiology. Braspen Journal. 2019;**34**(1):88-93

[40] Silva EF, Laste G, Torres RL, Hidalgo MPL, Stroher R, Torres ILS. Consumo de álcool e tabaco: Fator de risco para doença cardiovascular em população idosa do sul do Brasil. Revista Saúde e Desenvolvimento Humano. 2017;**5**(1):23-33

[41] Mantovani KCC et al. Poluentes do ar e internações devido a doenças cardiovasculares em São José do Rio Preto. Brasil Ciência & Saúde Coletiva. 2016;**21**(2):509-515

[42] Fioranelli M et al. Stress and inflammation in coronary artery disease: A review psycho neuroendocrine immunology based. Frontiers in Immunology. 2018;**9**(2031):1-15

[43] Askin L, Tanriverdi O, Askin HS. O Efeito da Doença de Coronavírus 2019 nas Doenças Cardiovasculares. Arquivos Brasileiros de Cardiologia. 2020;**114**(5):817-822

[44] Tseng F-Y, Lin W-Y, Lin C-C, et al. Subclinical hypothyroidism is associated with increased risk for all-cause and cardiovascular mortality in adults. Journal of the American College of Cardiology. 2012;**60**:730-737

[45] Bucharles BSE, Varela AM, Barberato SH, Filho RP. Avaliação e manejo da doença cardiovascular em pacientes com doença renal crônica. Journal Brasileiro de Nefrologia. 2010;**32**(1):120-127

[46] Santos IS et al. Atrial fibrillation diagnosis using ECG records and self-report in the community: Cross-sectional analysis from ELSA-brasil. Arquivos Brasileiros de Cardiologia. 2021;**117**(3):426-434

[47] Alraies MC, Eckman P. Adult heart transplant: Indications and outcomes. Journal of Thoracic Disease. 2014;**6**(8):1120-1128

[48] Antithrombotic Trialists' Collaboration. Collaborative

meta-analysis of randomized trials of antiplatelet therapy for prevention of death, myocardial infarction, and stroke in high risk patients. British Medical Journal. 2002;**324**(7329):71-86

[49] Cesar LA et al. Diretriz de Doença Coronária Estável. Arquivos Brasileiros de Cardiologia. 2014;**103**:1-59

[50] CURRENT-OASIS 7 Investigators, Mehta SR, Bassand JP, Chrolavicius S, Diaz R, Eikelboom JW, et al. Dose comparisons of clopidogrel and aspirin in acute coronary syndromes. The New England Journal of Medicine. 2010;**363**:930-942

[51] Steering Committee CAPRIE. A randomised, blinded, trial of clopidogrel versus aspirin in patients at risk of ischaemic events (CAPRIE). Lancet. 1996;**348**:1329-1339

[52] Serrano CV Jr, Soeiro AM, Leal TCAT, Godoy LC, Biselli B, Hata LA, et al. Statement on antiplatelet agents and anticoagulants in cardiology - 2019. Arquivos Brasileiros de Cardiologia. 2019;**113**(1):111-134

[53] Roe MT et al. TRILOGY ACS Investigators. Prasugrel versus clopidogrel for acute coronary syndromes without revascularization. The New England Journal of Medicine. 2012;**367**:1297-1309

[54] Wiviott SD, Braunwald E, McCabe CH, Montalescot G, Ruzyllo W, Gottlieb S, et al. Prasugrel versus clopidogrel in patients with acute coronary syndromes. The New England Journal of Medicine. 2007;**357**:2001-2015

[55] Zhang H, Yuan X, Zhang H, Chen S, Zhao Y, Hua K, et al. Efficacy of long-term beta-blocker therapy for secondary prevention of long-term outcomes after coronary artery bypass grafting surgery. Circulation. 2015;**131**:2194-2201

[56] Storey RF, Bliden KP, Ecob R, Karunakaran A, Butler K, Wei C, et al. Earlier recovery of platelet function after discontinuation of treatment with ticagrelor compared with clopidogrel in patients with high antiplatelet responses. Journal of Thrombosis and Haemostasis. 2011;**9**:1730-1737

[57] Vranckx P, Valgimigli M, Windecker S, Steg PG, Hamm C, Juni P, et al. Long-term ticagrelor monotherapy versus standard dual antiplatelet therapy followed by aspirin monotherapy in patients undergoing biolimus-eluting stent implantation: Rationale and design of the GLOBAL LEADERS trial. EuroIntervention. 2016;**12**:1239-1245

[58] Wallentin L et al. Biomarkers in relation to the effects of ticagrelor in comparison with clopidog-rel in non-ST-elevation acute coronary syndrome patients managed with or without in-hospital revascularization: A substudy from the prospective randomized platelet inhibition and patient outcomes (PLATO) trial. Circulation. 2014;**129**:293-303

[59] Valgimigli M et al. 2017 ESC focused update on dual antiplatelet therapy in coronary artery disease developed in collaboration with EACTS: The task force for dual antiplatelet therapy in coronary artery disease of the European Society of Cardiology (ESC) and of the European Association for Cardio-Thoracic Surgery (EACTS). European Heart Journal. 2018;**39**:213-260

[60] Agewall S et al. Expert position paper on the use of proton pump inhibitors in patients with cardiovascular disease and antithrombotic therapy. European Heart Journal. 2013;**34**:1708-1713

[61] Kirchhof P et al. 2016 ESC guidelines for the management of atrial fibrillation developed in collaboration

with EACTS. European Heart Journal. 2016;**37**:2893-2962

[62] Ohman EM et al. Clinically significant bleeding with low-dose rivaroxaban versus aspirin, in addition to P2Y12 inhibition, in acute coronary syndromes (GEMINI-ACS-1): A double-blind, multicentre, randomised trial. Lancet. 2017;**389**:1799-1808

[63] Mach F et al. 2019 ESC/EAS guidelines for the management of dyslipidaemias: Lipid modification to reduce cardiovascular risk. European Heart Journal. 2020;**41**:111-188

[64] Rosenson RS et al. Optimizing cholesterol treatment in patients with muscle complaints. Journal of the American College of Cardiology. 2017;**70**:1290-1301

[65] Ray KK, Stoekenbroek RM, Kallend D, et al. Effect of 1 or 2 doses of inclisiran on low-density lipoprotein cholesterol levels: One-year follow-up of the ORION-1 randomized clinical trial. JAMA Cardiology. 2019;**4**(11):1067-1075

[66] Radaelli G et al. O uso de inibidores da enzima conversora de angiotensina e sua relação com eventos no pósoperatório de cirurgia de revascularização miocárdica. Revista Brasileira de Cirurgia Cardiovascular. 2011;**26**(3):373-379

[67] Francisco YA, Bombig MTN. Tratamento da hipertensão arterial na insuficiência cardíaca. Revista Brasileira de Hipertensão. 2013;**20**(3):122-127

[68] Ponikowski P, Voors AA, Anker SD, Bueno H, Cleland JG, Coats AJ, et al. 2016 ESC guideline for the diagnosis and treatment of acute and chronic heart failure. European Heart Journal. 2016;**37**:2129-2200

[69] Poole-Wilson PA et al. Coronary disease trial investigating Outcome with nifedipine gastrointestinal therapeutic system investigators. Effect of long-acting nifedipine on mortality and cardiovascular morbidity in patients with stable angina requiring treatment (ACTION trial): Randomised controlled trial. Lancet. 2004;**364**:849-857

[70] McMurray JJ et al. Angiotensin-neprilysin inhibition versus enalapril in heart failure. The New England Journal of Medicine. 2014;**371**:993-1004

[71] Jouven X, Empana JP, Schwartz PJ, Desnos M, Courbon D, Ducimetiere P. Heart-rate profile during exercise as a predictor of sudden death. The New England Journal of Medicine. 2005;**352**:1951-1958

[72] Hwang D et al. Prognostic impact of betablocker dose after acute myocardial infarction. Circulation Journal. 2019;**83**:410-417

[73] Shu de F, Dong BR, Lin XF, Wu TX, Liu GJ. Long-term beta blockers for stable angina: Systematic review and meta-analysis. European Journal of Preventive Cardiology. 2012;**19**:330-341

[74] Werdan K, Ebelt H, Nuding S, Höpfner F, Hack G, Müller-Werdan U. Ivabradine in combination with beta-blocker improves symptoms and quality of life in patients with stable angina pectoris: Results from the Additions study. Clinical Research in Cardiology. 2012;**101**:365-373

[75] Pitt B, Ferreira JP, Zannad F. Mineralocorticoid receptor antagonists in patients with heart failure: Current experience and future perspectives. European Heart Journal - Cardiovascular Pharmacotherapy. 2017;**3**:48-57

[76] Pitt B et al. Eplerenone, a selective aldosterone blocker, in patients with left ventricular dysfunction after myocardial

infarction. The New England Journal of Medicine. 2003;**348**:1309-1321

[77] Lopaschuk GD, Verma S. Mechanisms of cardiovascular benefits of sodium glucose Co-transporter 2 (SGLT2) inhibitors: A state-of-the-art review. JACC: Basic to Translational Science. 2020;**5**(6):632-644

[78] Wanner C, Lachin JM, Inzucchi SE, et al. Empagliflozin and clinical outcomes in patients with type 2 diabetes mellitus, established cardiovascular disease, and chronic kidney disease. Circulation. 2018;**137**:119-129

[79] Packer M. Do sodium-glucose co-transporter-2 inhibitors prevent heart failure with a preserved ejection fraction by counterbalancing the effects of leptin? A novel hypothesis. Diabetes, Obesity & Metabolism. 2018;**20**(6):1361-1366

[80] Zinman B, Wanner C, Lachin JM, et al. For the EMPA-REG OUTCOME investigators: Empagliflozin, cardiovascular outcomes, and mortality in type 2 diabetes. The New England Journal of Medicine. 2015;**373**:2117-2128

[81] Wiviott SD, Raz I, Bonaca MP, et al. DECLARE–TIMI 58 Investigators. Dapagliflozin and cardiovascular outcomes in type 2 diabetes. The New England Journal of Medicine. 2019;**380**(4):347-357

[82] McCarthy CP, Mullins KV, Kerins DM. The role of trimetazidine in cardiovascular disease: Beyond an anti-anginal agent. European Heart Journal - Cardiovascular Pharmacotherapy. 2016;**2**:266-272

[83] Weisz G et al. Ranolazine in patients with incomplete revascularisation after percutaneous coronary intervention (RIVER-PCI): A multicentre, randomised, double-blind, placebo-controlled trial. Lancet. 2016;**387**:136-145

[84] Van Der Wal MHL, Jaarsma T. Adherence in heart failure in the elderly: Problem and possible solutions. International Journal of Cardiology. 2008;**125**:203-208

[85] Fonarrow GC et al. Factors identified as precipitating hospital admissions for heart failure and clinical outcomes: Findings for OPTIMIZE-HF. Archives of Internal Medicine. 2008;**168**(8):847-854

[86] Castro RA, Aliti GB, Linhares JC, Rabelo ER. Adesão ao tratamento de pacientes com insuficiência cardíaca em um hospital universitário. Revista Gaúcha de Enfermagem. 2010;**31**(2):225-231

[87] Schwartz BG, Kloner RA. Erectile dysfunction and cardiovascular disease. Circulation. 2011;**123**:98-101

[88] FMA F. A doença cardíaca, a insegurança e a disfunção sexual. Sociedade de Cardiologia do Estado do Rio de Janeiro. 2020;**13**(3):50-56

[89] Fonseca GWP, Santos MR, Souza FR, Alves MJNN. Testosterona e doença cardiovascular: do tratamento ao uso abusivo. A Sociedade de Cardiologia do Estado de São Paulo. 2019;**29**(4):393-399

[90] Santos MR, Dias RG, Laterza MC, Rondon MU, Braga AM, de Moraes Moreau RL, et al. Impaired post exercise heart rate recovery in anabolic steroid users. International Journal of Sports Medicine. 2013;**34**(10):931-935

[91] Yadav AK, Banerjee D, Lal A, Jha V. Vitamin D deficiency, CD4+CD28null cells and accelerated atherosclerosis in chronic kidney disease. Nephrology (Carlton, Vic.). 2012;**17**(6):575-581

[92] Junior FCM, Mandarino NR, Salgado JVL, Lages JS, Filho NS.

Deficiência de vitamina D: um novo fator de risco cardiovascular? Revista Brasileira de Cardiologia Invasiva. 2014;**27**(5):356-365

[93] Adams JS, Hewison M. Update in vitamin D. The Journal of Clinical Endocrinology and Metabolism. 2010;**95**(2):471-478

[94] Martins WA et al. Vacinação do cardiopata contra COVID-19: As razões da prioridade. Arquivos Brasileiros de Cardiologia. 2021;**116**(2):213-218

[95] Martins WA et al. Vacinação contra influenza e pneumococo na insuficiência cardíaca - Uma recomendação pouco aplicada. Arquivos Brasileiros de Cardiologia. 2011;**96**(3):240-245

[96] Harb SC, Marwick TH. Prognostic value of stress imaging after revascularization: A systematic review of stress echocardiography and stress nuclear imaging. American Heart Journal. 2014;**167**:7785

Chapter 7

Coronary Artery Bypass Grafting in High-Risk Patients: On-Pump Beating-Heart CABG

Antonio Nenna, Chiara Ferrisi, Antonio Salsano, Mario Lusini, Francesco Santini and Massimo Chello

Abstract

The tailored surgical approach in high-risk patients undergoing coronary artery bypass graft (CABG) still remains debated. Each classic operative technique has strengths and limitations: on-pump CABG entails the use of cardiopulmonary bypass and cardioplegic arrest, while off-pump "beating heart" CABG is technically challenging and might pose problems in case of preoperative hemodynamic impairment or recent myocardial infarction. The hybrid approach of on-pump beating-heart CABG (OPBHC) has been proposed over the years as an acceptable trade-off in cases of severe complications caused by cardioplegic arrest or manipulation of the heart. This chapter intends to summarize the available literature about OPBHC, considering both original contributions and secondary research papers, trying to define operative indications and future perspectives. OPBHC, preventing hemodynamic deterioration while sustaining adequate end-organ perfusion, has been gradually recognized as an effective technique for performing surgical revascularization in high-risk patients, such as those presenting with acute coronary syndrome, cardiogenic shock, or severe left ventricular dysfunction. In selected cases, OPBHC reduces in-hospital mortality and decreases the risk of perioperative complications such as myocardial ischemia or stroke and should be considered a valid alternative to conventional off-pump and on-pump CABG techniques. OPBHC should be in the armamentarium of the next-generation cardiac surgeon.

Keywords: coronary artery bypass grafting, left ventricular dysfunction, myocardial revascularization, off-pump beating-heart, off-pump, on-pump, cardiopulmonary bypass

1. Introduction

Coronary artery disease is a common pathological condition that is increasingly undermining people's health. This disease can be treated with different targeted strategies, such as medical therapy, percutaneous revascularization (PCI), or coronary bypass surgery. These treatments are often complementary, and they should not be seen as mere alternatives. However, patients with symptoms refractory to medical therapy, left main or triple vessels disease, or complex coronary anatomy not suitable for PCI (or failed PCI) require an inevitable surgery.

Regarding coronary bypass surgeries, there are several methods and techniques have dramatically evolved since the late 1970s. Coronary artery bypass grafting (CABG) is commonly performed for patients with stenosis exceeding a 70% reduction in vessel diameter, delivering blood to the distal coronary artery beyond a stenosis.

There are two different surgical techniques of CABG that are commonly used: on-pump "conventional" CABG and off-pump "beating heart" CABG. The use of cardiopulmonary bypass (CPB) and cardioplegia are the main characteristics that distinguish these two types of surgery. There are several pros and cons to using these two surgical techniques, which should be evaluated carefully before assessing which method is more effective and suitable in different cases.

The cardiopulmonary bypass carries several risks, and in 1% of cases, it leads to cerebral damage due to intracerebral bleeding, embolization of microbubbles, arterial debris, or inadequate cerebral perfusion. Moreover, it brings the activation of several systematic inflammatory mechanisms, with cytokine release and complement activation. Coagulopathy and hemolysis could also occur. All these processes can be the main factors for post-bypass patients in developing pulmonary and renal dysfunctions.

In the on-pump surgery, as mentioned previously, the use of cardioplegic arrest is the main characteristic of this technique. Cardioplegia is a solution made of electrolytic, especially high doses of potassium, which causes heart arrest in diastole. Cardioplegia is typically delivered at a temperature of 4–6°C and via a crystalloid solution or one derived from the patient's own blood. Coronary arteries are perfused by the cardioplegia via the aortic root or directly via the coronary artery ostia, or retrogradely via a catheter placed in the coronary sinus. Cardioplegia, combined with hypothermia, guarantees a safe period of cardiac arrest in which the surgeon will perform the graft.

Contrarily, during an off-pump surgery, the coronary bypass is performed without the use of any cardioplegia, hence on a beating heart. This alternative surgery is commonly used in specific cases, such as in the presence of a markedly calcified ascending aorta. However, this type of surgery does not avoid cardiac risks, in particular when hemodynamic instability arises from the surgical manipulation and immediate conversion to the on-pump conventional CABG is needed.

Considering the risks of both techniques, a new hybrid approach has been studied and tested to overcome the limitations of each technique trying to gather benefits from both, and the dichotomy between "on-pump" versus "off-pump" CABG has been made more complex by the introduction of the beating heart on-pump CABG (OPBHC). OPBHC technique was introduced in the mid-1990s, and it combined the main characteristics of the previous two methods, providing hemodynamic stability with the CPB without aortic cross-clamp and cardioplegic cardiac arrest, preserving native coronary blood flow.

Literature search was performed through PubMed, Web of Science, Scopus, and Cochrane database from their inception up to July 2023 using the following search keywords in various combinations: "myocardial infarction", "myocardial revascularization", "on-pump beating-heart", "coronary artery bypass graft"/"CABG", "cardiogenic shock", "left ventricular dysfunction". We also reviewed references of prior randomized trials, prospective/retrospective cohort studies, systematic reviews, meta-analyses, and references from selected articles. All papers describing post-operative outcomes after on-pump beating-heart CABG were included, as this was considered the "intervention". The "comparators" were on-pump CABG or off-pump CABG when compared to OPBHC. Outcomes included early mortality, postoperative complications, and time-to-event outcomes. Editorials, opinion articles, and repeat publications of the same data set were excluded from the quantitative synthesis.

2. Off-pump CABG vs. on-pump CABG vs. "on-pump beating heart CABG" (OPBHC)

Despite the flourishing literature after its introduction, OPBHC still remains considered a non-valuable option by many surgeons in the real-world scenario, who are afraid of its complications. However, the literature produced a considerable amount of evidence to draw objective conclusions.

A recent study by Jiang et al. [1] studied the main pros and cons of using off-pump CABG vs. the use of OPBHC by analyzing the rate of early mortality and long-term survival of patients. The study enrolled a total of 5615 patients, of which less than one-third underwent OPBHC, and the remaining were treated with off-pump CABG. The main conclusion was that no significant statistical differences have been found, in terms of early mortality and long-term survival rates, among the patients treated with these two techniques. The use of CPB, in both conventional on-pump and OPBHC, can lead to some complications, such as renal failure, strokes, arrhythmia, coagulopathy, platelet dysfunction, and increased drainage or blood loss, increasing postoperative morbidity and mortality. Hence, for some patients, the off-pump CABG might be a suitable surgery. However, patients with hemodynamic instability cannot tolerate prolonged heart manipulation, requiring CPB support. In these cases, the study suggested that the OPBHC can play a crucial role, providing more effective hemodynamic support than off-pump CABG but with a shorter CPB time than conventional on-pump CABG.

Another study by Wang et al. [2] analyzed the benefits of the OPBHC technique vs. the conventional on-pump CABG in high-risk patients. The main conclusions were that OPBHC surgery had lower mortality and similar long-term survival rates than conventional on-pump CABG. Moreover, the study suggests that the OPBHC technique leads to a lower risk of renal failure, thanks to the avoidance of both systemic hypothermia and hypoperfusion of end-organ and the shorter CPB time. This is explained by the fact that in conventional on-pump CABG, the prolonged use of CPB leads to acute kidney injuries. All of this is confirmed by the evidence that a higher number of patients undergone conventional on-pump CABG require hemodialysis than the patients undergone OPBHC surgeries.

Other studies [3, 4] highlighted that OPBHC surgery could lead to a significant acute kidney injury due to higher right atrial pressure, higher distended heart, less venous return from the kidney, and less glomerular filtration function than off and on-pump CABG. The study suggests that the use of left ventricular venting in the conventional on-pump decompresses the heart, lowering the venue's return from kidney. Instead, the off-pump surgery guarantees renal protection thanks to pulsatile flow and normal kidney perfusion pressure. Summarizing data from the literature, factors that might be associated with potential benefits for the OPBHC approach are shown in **Table 1**. As no randomized evidence is available, recommendations about OPBHC remain based on expert opinions.

Considering procedural details, heart positioning during OPBHC can be tailored to vessel exposition without compromising hemodynamics, as perfusion is

Preoperative factors
Acute coronary syndrome
Cardiogenic shock
Early graft failure
Emergency surgery
Redo surgery
Left ventricular dysfunction
Intraoperative factors
Difficult-to-approach coronary targets using off-pump technique
High risk of complications using off-pump technique
Intramyocardial vessels
Unstable hemodynamics
Poor-quality coronary targets
Diffused calcification
Small diameter

Table 1.
Factors associated with potential benefit from OPBHC approach.

guaranteed by cardiopulmonary bypass. In general, central cannulation is performed (arterial cannula in ascending aorta and venous cannula in right atrium). The graft sequence is similar to off-pump CABG, with the left anterior descending artery being revascularized first (in general with the left internal thoracic artery), followed by obtuse marginal vessels and a posterior descending artery or right circumflex artery. Composite grafts (i.e., Y-graft) can be performed before or after distal anastomosis, depending on the surgeon's preference. A heart can be moved freely during OPBHC, and stabilization can be achieved with pericardial stitches and epicardial stabilizer to improve exposure. In our clinical practice, the use of an intracoronary shunt to minimize heart ischemia is mandatory, with no other arterial occlude device (e.g., loop above and below the anastomosis site).

3. OPBHC: indications and results

OPBHC might be an alternative method useful in high-risk conditions, such as cardiogenic shock, reduced LVEF, or redo-CABG. Several observational studies and meta-analyses have been carried out between 2000 and 2022, but specific and official guidelines for OPBHC are still missing from international societies. In fact, this technique is still underused across the world, but in trained centers with more advanced testing phases, the results are promising and positive.

A study by Zhu et al. [5, 6] has demonstrated that the level of success of this technique is highly correlated to the level of knowledge and experience in using it. The study reviewed the ANZSCTS (Australian and New Zealand Society of Cardiac and Thoracic Surgery) database, in which only 1.3% of patients across Australia with emergent CABG within 7 days after acute myocardial injury underwent OPBHC surgery. By contrast, the same study revealed that in Japan, the same technique was performed in 24% of the cases, highlighting more powerful results than those in Australia on OPBHC. Hence, the choice of which method is more suitable primarily depends on surgical expertise, the patient's hemodynamical status, and comorbidities.

3.1 OPBHC in specific setting: acute myocardial infarction and cardiogenic shock

Acute myocardial infarction (MI) is an emergent situation treated with percutaneous procedures (PCI). In case of unfavorable coronary anatomy for percutaneous approach or failure/complications of percutaneous interventions or myocardial ischemia refractory to medical therapy, urgent CABG should be performed. Yet, a conventional on-pump CABG might deteriorate cardiac function as the use of cardioplegia delivered into an infarcted myocardium could lead to a high risk of ischemia–reperfusion syndrome. On the other hand, off-pump CABG might not be a safe technique because of hemodynamic instability that requires a higher dose of inotropes and vasopressors, which could lead to end-organ damage. Heart manipulation or compression needed for bypass grafting might cause refractory hypotension or arrhythmias, leading to an emergent intraoperative conversion to on-pump CABG as a life-saving procedure. In this case, an emergent conversion to an on-pump CABG could lead to up to a sevenfold increased risk of mortality and a 40% crude mortality rate [7].

In this context, the OPBHC could be a suitable solution (**Table 2**). The CPB reduces ventricular volume loading, allowing heart mobilization without significant consequences on coronary flow or myocardial stability. In addition, this approach might guarantee grafting of the lateral and inferior wall of the heart, performing a higher rate of complete revascularization than in off-pump CABG procedures. Cardiogenic shock after acute MI occurs in 10–20% of cases, and it is the leading cause of in-hospital mortality. Despite PCI being the targeted therapy in cardiogenic shock after acute MI, GUSTO-1, and SCHOCK trials [7, 14] reveal that CABG had comparable mortality rates to PCI in patients with complex coronary artery disease anatomy and high-risk profile. In addition, CABG guarantees a higher rate of complete revascularization (87% in CABG vs. 23% in PCI) [7, 14]. In an urgent situation, OPBHC avoids cardioplegic arrest and aortic cross-clamping, provides end-organ perfusion, thanks to CPB, and reduces the injection of inotrope drugs. The Rastan et al. [12] study showed that hospital mortality between conventional on-pump CABG and OPBHC was similar ($p = 0.8$). The study included patients with stable hemodynamics at admission, performing in 48.4% conventional on-pump CABG and in 51.6% OPBHC. Moreover, the study observed that when an OPBHC was performed, despite the use of an emergent conversion to CPB, the in-hospital mortality of patients with cardiogenic shock at admission was reduced ($p = 0.48$). The Rastan et al. [12] study also highlighted that in OPBHC surgeries, the use of postoperative intra-aortic balloon pump (IABP) and inotrope drugs after CABG is reduced. In addition, the study showed that the shorter duration of CBP during OPBHC, increasing myocardial perfusion and reducing myocardial stunning, leads to a reduction in myocardial infarction after surgery.

3.2 Left ventricular dysfunction

The best CABG strategy in patients with poor left ventricular ejection fraction (LVEF) is still debated. Data [1, 6, 7] showed that on-pump CABG carries additional risk in patients with impaired LVEF, mainly because of cardioplegic arrest and related biventricular dysfunction. The results of Prifti et al. [15] underlined how the use of OPHBC may be a successful alternative to CABG with cardioplegic arrest. However, off-pump surgery may lead to incomplete revascularization and intraoperative hemodynamic deterioration. Xia et al. [16] study showed that patients with impaired

Author	Year	Design	Control group	Patients	Risk scores	Short term mortality	Other short-term outcomes	Long term mortality	Other long-term outcomes
Zhu et al. [5]	2019	PS	On-pump CABG	77 vs. 154	EuroSCORE 1 log: 12.3 vs. 14.9, p = 0.98	Similar (11.7% vs. 10.4%, p = 0.85)	Similar MACCEs (22.1% vs. 24.7%, p = 0.84); increased rate of incomplete revascularization (19.5% vs. 9.7%, p = 0.03); slightly reduced left internal mammary artery use (75.3% vs. 84.4%, p = 0.08)	Similar (64.8% [39.4–82.4%] vs. 63.6% [50.5%–74.3%], p = 0.89) (12 years)	NA
Tsai et al. [8]	2012	RS	Off-pump CABG; on-pump CABG	48 OPBHC 56 off-pump 82 on-pump	EuroSCORE 1 log: OPBHC 11.4%, off-pump 8.4%, on-pump 9.9% (p = 0.01)	Reduced 4.2% OPBHC vs. 5.4% off-pump vs. 8.5% on-pump (p = 0.57)	Hospital days 13.1 OPBHC vs. 12.6 off-pump vs. 16.5 on-pump (p = 0.001)	2-, 4-, 6- and 8-year survival rates(%): 70.1, 66.7, 65.1, 65.1 on-pump; 91.1, 81.4, 76.5, 73.8 off-pump; 93.7, 87.0, 87.0, 87.0 OPBHC (p = 0.023)	Similar freedom from cardiac events
Munos et al. [9]	2011	RS	Off-pump CABG; mini-CEC; on-pump CABG	51 OPBHC 57 off-pump 51 mini-CEC 55 on-pump	EuroSCORE 1 log >20% in 61% of patients OPBHC, 67% off-pump, 59% mini-CEC, 57% on-pump (p = 0.01)	Similar (OPBHC (2%) compared with the other groups (4.9%), p = 0.36)	Average length of ICU stay 2.53 days vs. 2.16 OPBHC, (p = 0.02); increased complete revascularization (95% vs. 89% for off-pump CABG)	NA	NA

Author	Year	Design	Control group	Patients	Risk scores	Short term mortality	Other short-term outcomes	Long term mortality	Other long-term outcomes
Miyahara et al. [10]	2008	RS	On-pump CABG	38 vs. 23	EuroSCORE 1 log: 9.9 ± 1.6 vs. 9.0 ± 1.6, p = 0.04; preoperative IABP 78.9% vs. 43.5%, p = 0.005	Reduced (2.6% vs. 21.7%, p = 0.046)	Similar graft patency (98.5% vs. 95.7%, p = 0.090); reduced number of distal anastomoses (2.0 ± 0.7 vs. 2.9 ± 0.9, p = 0.001); similar IABP use (0% vs. 3%, p = 0.220); shorter CPB time (126 ± 36 vs. 185 ± 49 min, p = 0.001)	NA	NA
Ferrari et al. [11]	2008	RS	None	25	EuroSCORE 1 log>8 in most patients	8%	Hospital stay 12.0 ± 6.7 days; complete revascularization 92%; IABP use 11%	95.6% (year)	NA
Rastan et al. [12]	2006	RS	On-pump CABG	157 vs. 374 (stable hemodynamics)	EuroSCORE 1 log: 9.6 vs. 8.0, p = 0.01; EuroSCORE > 20: 24.8% vs. 13.9%, p = 0.004	Similar (5.7% vs. 8.6%, p = 0.08)	Reduced hospital stay (10.4 ± 6.8 vs. 12.6 ± 8.2, p = 0.015); increased incomplete revascularization (17.8% vs. 10.7%, p = 0.032); reduced inotropic support (36.3% vs. 52.1%, p < 0.001); reduced reoperation for bleeding (0.6% vs. 4.8%, p = 0.020)	Similar (84.1% vs. 82.1%, p = 0.791) (4 years)	Similar freedom from adverse events (78.2% vs. 74.5%, p = 0.511); similar repeated revascularization rates (7.9% vs. 5.0%, p = 0.74) (4 years)

Author	Year	Design	Control group	Patients	Risk scores	Short term mortality	Other short-term outcomes	Long term mortality	Other long-term outcomes
Rastan et al. [12]	2006	RS	On-pump CABG	83 vs. 24 (cardiogenic shock)	EuroSCORE 1 log: 25.5 vs. 26.2, p = 0.69	Reduced (19.3% vs. 33.3%, p = 0.048)	Reduced stroke (9.6% vs. 33.3%, p = 0.009); reduced atrial fibrillation (39.8% vs. 62.5%, p = 0.041); reduced inotropic support (65.1% vs. 87.5%, p = 0.049) Similar incomplete revascularization rate (12.0% vs. 20.8%, p = 0.275)	Similar (60.3% vs. 44.5%, p = 0.109) (4 years)	Similar freedom from adverse events 56.4% vs. 36.1%, p = 0.079 (4 years)
Izumi et al. [13]	2006	RS	On-pump CABG	15 vs. 16	NA	Similar (13.3% vs. 31.3%, p = 0.39)	Reduced renal failure (13.3% vs. 64.3%, p = 0.009) similar number of anastomosis (2.3 vs. 2.5, p = 0.202)	NA	NA

AKI: acute kidney injury; CABG: coronary artery bypass grafting; PS: propensity-score adjusted/matched study; RS: retrospective study; REG: registry; RCT: randomized controlled trial; AMI: acute myocardial infarction; MACE: major adverse cardiovascular events; NA: not applicable; NS: not significant; OPBHC: on-pump beating heart coronary artery bypass grafting. Data are referred as OPBHC group versus control group unless otherwise indicated (see table for details). Adapted from Dominici et al. [7].

Table 2.
Summary of the evidence for OPBHC in patients with acute myocardial infarction, cardiogenic shock, and chronic kidney disease.

LVEF, undergoing OPHBC or off-pump surgeries, have the same in-hospital mortality rate ($p = 0.741$). Yet, in c3.9% of the cases, an emergent conversion from off-pump to OPHBC was needed due to hemodynamic instability or ventricular fibrillation, therefore increasing the mortality rate (reaching around 40%). A recent study by Wang et al. [2] highlighted that, even if in some patients, an emergent conversion from off-pump to OPBHC was required, no differences were found in in-hospital mortality between the two groups (OPBHC vs. off-pump CABG—$p = 0.973$).

OPHBC had better short-term outcomes, showing a lower rate of early mortality, lower use of IABP, and lower incidence of stroke than on-pump CABG (**Table 3**). However, the long-term outcomes have shown a clear preference for OPBHC due to incomplete revascularization. Conventional on-pump CABG had higher rates of complete revascularization than OPBHC. On the other hand, off-pump CABG had a lower rate than OPBHC. An analysis of Darwazah et al. [18] showed that OPBHC was the surgical procedure more common than off-pump CABG in redo CABG (13% vs. 3% $p = 0.025$). According to a similar degree of coronary disease, OPBHC guaranteed an increasing number of distal grafts ($p = 0.002$) and complete revascularization. The main difference between the two procedures was the hemodynamic instability during cardiac manipulation that prevented complete revascularization in patients who underwent off-pump surgery.

3.3 OPBHC in unselected population

There are several studies showing that the use of OPBHC as an ordinary revascularization strategy reduces the level of in-hospital mortality (**Table 4**). This was confirmed by the Mizutani et al. [23] study, which found that the level of in-hospital mortality among low-risk patients was lower in the OPBHC group ($p < 0.001$), adding that the elimination of cardioplegic arrest might play a crucial role in case of deteriorated hemodynamic.

Furthermore, other studies (like the one of Antunes et al. [21]) have confirmed this thesis, showing that a high level of trained staff, combined with adequate preoperative care, can improve the outcome by lowering the level of mortality. Contrarily, a study by Kim et al. [20] highlighted that the level of mortality and postoperative complications among the OPBHC and on-pump CABG groups were similar.

3.4 OPBHG: results from secondary research and meta-analysis

One of the most common and feared postoperative complications after CABG is stroke, which mainly occurs when calcifications along the aorta embolize in brain vessels. During conventional on-pump CABG, two procedures might lead to postoperative stroke: aortic cannulation and aortic cross-clamping. According to this scenario, off-pump CABG represents the best surgical technique in patients with markedly calcified ascending aorta or in patients with a history of cerebrovascular events. In particular, off-pump CABG, with a no-touch approach, avoids aortic side-clamping, and it guarantees a significant reduction in neurological events. This issue has been carefully investigated in secondary research as it might be one of the most peculiar indications for OPBHC (**Table 5**).

The most recent metanalysis [1, 6, 7, 24] showed that postoperative stroke rate is similar between patients who underwent off-pump CABG and OPBHC. These data [7] suggest that the only aortic cannulation procedure might not affect cerebral disease after surgery. However, the dynamics of aortic side-clamping for proximal

Author	Year	Design	Control group	Patients	Risk scores	Short term mortality	Other short-term outcomes	Long term mortality	Other long-term outcomes
Wang et al. [2]	2019	RS	Off-pump CABG	44 vs. 68	EuroSCORE 1 log: 7.52 vs. 7.68, p = 0.77	Similar (4.5% vs. 4.4%, p = 0.973)	40% mortality rate for conversion; greater number of grafts (3.74 ± 0.84 vs. 3.36 ± 0.80, p < 0.001)	Similar data not shown, p = 0.674, mean follow up of 38.9 ± 16.7 months	Reduced MACEs data not shown, p = 0.049, mean follow up of 38.9 ± 16.7 months
Xia et al. [16]	2017	RS	Off-pump CABG	88 vs. 128	EuroSCORE 1 log>6: 50% vs. 47%, p = 0.782; all patients with LVEF <35%; increased left ventricular end-diastolic diameter in OPBHC(66.8 ± 6.0 vs. 64.7 ± 5.9, p = 0.013)	Similar (3.4% vs. 4.7%, p = 0.741)	40% mortality rate for conversion; higher number of grafts (3.7 ± 0.8 vs. 2.8 ± 0.6, p < 0.001); higher pre-discharge LVEF(35.6 ± 2.9 vs. 34.8 ± 3.3, p = 0.034	NA	NA
Erkut et al. [17]	2013	RS	On-pump CABG	65 vs. 66	NA	Reduced (3.1% vs. 21.2%, p = 0.001)	Reduced postoperative infarction (1.5% vs. 16.7%, p = 0.012)	Similar 77% vs. 70%, p > 0.05 (18 months)	NA
Darwazah et al. [18]	2010	RS	off-pump CABG	39 vs. 98	EuroSCORE 1 log: 14.1 vs. 12.2, p = 0.443	Similar (8% vs. 6%, p = 0.712)	Increased complete revascularization rate (72% vs. 46%, p = 0.015); increased number of distal anastomosis (2.2 ± 0.7 vs. 1.7 ± 0.7, p = 0.002)	NA	NA
Pegg et al. [19]	2008	RCT	On-pump CABG	25 vs. 25	EuroSCORE 1 log: 12 ± 10 vs. 8 ± 5, p = 0.079	Similar (4% vs. 0%, p = 0.31)	Similar MACEs 12% vs. 4%, p = 0.30	NA	NA

DOI: http://dx.doi.org/10.5772/intechopen.115054

Author	Year	Design	Control group	Patients	Risk scores	Short term mortality	Other short-term outcomes	Long term mortality	Other long-term outcomes
Prifti et al. [15]	2000	RS	On-pump CABG	107 vs. 191	NA	Similar (6.5 vs. 10%, p = 0.318)	Reduced perioperative infarction (4.7% vs. 13%, p = 0.034), renal dysfunction(29% vs. 41%, p = 0.05), ultrafiltration(5.6% vs. 15.7%, p = 0.017), bleeding >1000 mL(9% vs. 21.4%, p = 0.012)	Similar mortality rates at 1, 3 and 5 years of follow-up (p = NS)	Similar reoperation rates at follow-up (p = NS)

AKI: acute kidney injury; CABG: coronary artery bypass grafting; PS: propensity-score adjusted/matched study; RS: retrospective study; REG: registry; RCT: randomized controlled trial; AMI: acute myocardial infarction; MACE: major adverse cardiovascular events; NA: not applicable; NS: not significant; OPBHC: on-pump beating heart coronary artery bypass grafting. Data are referred as OPBHC group versus control group unless otherwise indicated (see table for details). Adapted from Dominici et al. [7].

Table 3.
Summary of the evidence for OPBHG in patients with left ventricular dysfunction.

Author	Year	Design	Control group	Patients	Short term mortality	Other short-term outcomes	Long term mortality	Other long-term outcomes
Phothikun et al. [3]	2023	RS	On-pump CABG and off-pump CABG	2028	Similar	Similar rate of cardiac index (p = 0.158)	Similar 10-years survival (80.5% vs. 75.9% vs. 73.7%)	OPBHG: reduced rate in MACE (HR 0.52; p = 0.04) and mortality (HR = 0.33; p = 0.01)
Kim et al. [20]	2018	RS	On-pump CABG	254 vs. 391 (173 vs. 173 propensity score-matched)	Similar (1.2% vs. 0%, p = 0.478)	Similar rate of AKI (5.9% vs. 0.8%, p = 0.001); similar rate of dialysis (4.6% vs. 1.2%, p = 0.109)	Similar (3.0% vs. 2.8%, p = 0.506)	Similar (all MACEs: 4.0% vs. 3.5%, p = 0.382)
Antunes et al. [21]	2015	RS	None	8515	0.7%	Stroke 2.6%, AKI 18.9%, myocardial infarction 2.5%	NA	NA
Narayan et al. [22]	2010	RCT	On-pump CABG	40 vs. 41	Similar (none)	NA	Similar 5-years survival (HR 0.62, 95% CI 0.15–2.59)	NA
Mizutani et al. [23]	2007	RS	On-pump CABG	114 vs. 114	Reduced (2.6% vs. 9.6%, p < 0.001)	Decreased rate of complete revascularization (42.1% vs. 77.2%, p < 0.001)	NA	NA

AKI: acute kidney injury; CABG: coronary artery bypass grafting; PS: propensity-score adjusted/matched study; RS: retrospective study; REG: registry; RCT: randomized controlled trial; AMI: acute myocardial infarction; MACE: major adverse cardiovascular events; NA: not applicable; NS: not significant; OPBHC: on-pump beating heart coronary artery bypass grafting. Data are referred as OPBHC group versus control group unless otherwise indicated (see table for details). Adapted from Dominici et al. [7].

Table 4.
Summary of the evidence for OPBHG in unselected patients.

Study	Year	Studies	Patients	Population	Short term mortality	Other short-term outcomes	Long term outcomes
Hwang et al. [24]	2022	19 (1 RCT)	4320 on-pump CABG vs. 5559 off-pump CABG vs. 1962 OPBHC	9 studies with high-risk patients (AMI)	Lower rate in off-pump CABG vs. OPBHC (OR 0.50; 95% CI 0.20–1.57)	Similar rate of stroke, AKI, and length of intensive care unit in off-pump CABG and OPBHC vs. on-pump CABG; Lower rate of myocardial infarction in off-pump CABG vs. on-pump CABG (OR 0.60; 95% CI 0.38–0.93; p = 0.02); lower risk of reoperation for bleeding in off-pump CABG vs. on-pump CABG (OR 0.54; 95% CI 0.37–0.80; p = 0.002)	NA
Wang et al. [6]	2021	24 (3 RCT)	1847 OPBHC vs. 5015 on-pump-CABG	9 studies with high-risk patients	Higher in on-pump CABG (OR 1.45; 95% CI 1.09–1.93; p = 0.01)	Higher risk of myocardial infarction in on-pump CABG (OR 2.60; 95% CI 1.41 to 4.78; p = 0.002); Higher risk of LOS in on-pump CABG (OR 2.56; 95% CI 1.55–4.23; p < 0.001); higher risk of AKI in on-pump CABG (OR 1.84;95% CI 1.38–2.44; p < 0.01); similar rate of hemodialysis (OR 1.23; 95% CI 0.74 to 2.12; p = 0.41); similar rate of incomplete revascularization (OR 0.65; 95% CI 0.40–1.05; p = 0.08)	Similar mortality (HR 1.08; 95% CI 0.81–1.43)
Jiang et al. [1]	2021	18 (5 RCT)	1548 OPBHC vs. 4067 off-pump CABG	18 studies with pairwise comparison	Similar (OR 1.28; 95% CI:0.91–0.80; p = 0.16)	Higher risk of stroke in OPBHC (OR 1767; 95% CI: 1.08–2.58; p = 0.02); similar heterogeneity of AKI (p = 0.09); lower risk of arrhythmias in off-pump CABG (OR 1.30; 95% CI: 1.06–1.6; p = 0.001); lower risk of incomplete revascularization in OPBHC (OR 0.67; 95% CI:0.49–0.92; p = 0.01); Higher risk of blood loss in OPHBC (CI 42.94–180.18; p = 0.001); Lower rate of distal anastomoses in off-pump CABG (CI 0.29 to 0.61; p < 0.00001)	Similar mortality (HR 0.86, 95% CI: 0.51–1.45; p = 0.57)

Study	Year	Studies	Patients	Population	Short term mortality	Other short-term outcomes	Long term outcomes
Dominici et al. [7]	2020	17 (2 RCT)	2331 OPBHC versus on-pump CABG; 677 OPBHC versus off-pump CABG	17 studies (12 on-pump CABG and 5 off-pump CABG) with pairwise comparison	Reduced (RR 0.59, 95% CI 0.36–0.97)	Reduced postoperative stroke (RR 0.60, 95% CI 0.39–0.91); reduced postoperative intra-aortic balloon pump use (RR 0.56, 95% CI 0.31–1.01); myocardial infarction (RR 0.48, 95% CI 0.22–1.07)	Lower risk of incomplete revascularization in OPBHC vs. off-pump CABG (RR 0.53, 95% CI 0.33–0.87). Higher risk of incomplete revascularization in OPBHC vs. on-pump CABG (RR 1.71, 95% CI 1.23–2.39)
Ueki et al. [25]	2016	14 (2 RCT)	884 OPBHC 1156 on-pump conventional CABG	Eight studies with high-risk patients (acute coronary syndrome, reduced LVEF, dialysis, EuroSCORE>9); 67.4% high predicted operative risk	Reduced (OR 0.55, 95% CI 0.38–0.81, $p = 0.008$)	Reduced myocardial infarction(OR 0.29, $p = 0.001$); reduced low cardiac output syndrome (OR 0.33, $p < 0.001$) reduced renal failure requiring hemodialysis (OR 0.36, $p < 0.001$); reduced reoperation for bleeding (OR 0.53, $p = 0.027$); similar number of grafts (WMD −0.12, $p = 0.30$); similar rates of incomplete revascularization (OR 1.77, $p = 0.15$); similar incidence of stroke (OR 0.64, $p = 0.089$)	NA

DOI: http://dx.doi.org/10.5772/intechopen.115054

Study	Year	Studies	Patients	Population	Short term mortality	Other short-term outcomes	Long term outcomes
Chaudhry et al. [26]	2015	13 (2 RCT)	937 OPBHC 2993 on-pump conventional CABG	83.6% unselected population, a high-risk subgroup was not specifically evaluated	Similar (OR 0.60, 95% CI 0.32–1.14, $p = 0.12$)	Reduced postoperative myocardial infarction (OR 0.32, $p = 0.03$); reduced IABP use (OR 0.51, $p = 0.04$); reduced CPB time (WMD −13.5, $p = 0.03$); similar number of grafts (WMD −0.20, $p = 0.61$); similar incidence of stroke (OR 0.85, $p = 0.54$); similar risk of renal failure (OR 0.49, $p = 0.20$); similar length of stay (WMD −2.71, $p = 0.08$)	Similar mortality (OR 0.65, 95% CI 0.22–1.88, $p = 0.43$)

OR: odds ratio; WMD: weighted mean difference. NA: not applicable. Data are referred as OPBHC group versus control group. Adapted from Dominici et al. [7].

Table 5.
Summary of the evidence for OPBHG: Secondary research and meta-analysis.

anastomosis are quite different. The OPBHC could lead to a proximal anastomosis in a "softer" aortic lateral clamping due to rapid on-demand hypotension achieved by CPB, while in off-pump CABG, the same procedure leads to a more traumatic side-clamping.

Also, considering short-term outcomes, recent studies are pointing out that a reduced risk of mortality of OPBHC is performed in selected patients (with high preoperative risk) [7, 25], while previous findings in unselected patients might have diluted the benefits [26].

Based on these results, OPBHC was shown to be associated with reduced postoperative mortality and complications (mainly driven by reduced stroke and reduced myocardial infarction) than conventional revascularization and might be suggested as a valid alternative in high-risk patients. However, considering the significant differences in inclusion criteria, future work should focus on registries and multicenter RCTs to definitely assess the benefits of OPBHC.

4. Gaps in evidence

Although several studies have been done on the OPBHC, there are still several aspects to be analyzed in order to have a clear overview of the benefits and implications of using it.

One aspect that would need to be further investigated is the optimal level of perfusion pressure during OPBHC. A low level of perfusion pressure might increase the risk of hypoperfusion in the distal and subendocardial territories, as low perfusion pressure might lead to flow competition and insufficient native coronary artery blood flow. Evidence from metanalysis [1, 6, 7, 24] suggests that a mean pressure between 70 and 80 mmHg could be an optimal level but due to few observations within the sample, more studies should be performed on this topic.

Another risk for patients undergoing an OPBHC is manipulation-induced aortic insufficiency. In fact, the hemodynamic stability of the patient could be affected by an excessive acute aortic regurgitation when the blood flow comes from the aortic cannula. Further investigations on this risk are needed to better assess the OPBHC technique.

In emergency situations, surgeons usually prefer to use vein grafts rather than arterial conduits as this procedure is faster and less complex. However, the use of vein grafts could affect the long-term outcomes of CABG. Hence, more studies should evaluate if long-term outcomes are affected by the type of graft conduits used (vein or arterial) in the OPBHC setting, as several published researches have been conducted for conventional on-pump CABG.

Another aspect to be further investigated is the level of surgeons' experience, as this might weigh on the overall valuation of the OPBHC technique. For example, emergency conversion to CPB is usually followed by a higher risk of mortality. The use of OPBHC could reduce this risk if it is combined with a well-trained surgeon and anesthesiologic team.

Finally, further investigations should evaluate the risk associated with the use of OPBHC or PCI for the revascularization of left ventricular. In fact, OPBHC surgeries are associated with a high level of risk for patients but with good graft patency over time. On the other hand, PCI techniques require more advanced and difficult procedures to guarantee complete revascularization without avoiding subsequent myocardial injuries.

5. Conclusion

In conclusion, for high-risk patients, such as those with acute coronary syndrome, cardiogenic shock or with left ventricular dysfunction, the OPBHC seems to be a valid alternative to the off-pump and on-pump CABG techniques, reducing early mortality and decreasing the risk of postoperative complications such as myocardial ischemia or stroke. In particular, the OPBHC could provide an acceptable trade-off in cases of severe complications caused by cardioplegic arrest or manipulation of the heart. Although this technique is still in a rising phase, there are several studies and secondary research supporting its benefits, and we advocate its introduction in future guidelines for revascularization. However, more analyses are needed to develop a common consensus to overcome the blind spots (such as its long-term clinical impacts) that are preventing its adoption as a recognized technique worldwide.

Conflict of interest

The authors declare no conflict of interest.

Notes/thanks/other declarations

None.

Author details

Antonio Nenna[1]*, Chiara Ferrisi[1], Antonio Salsano[2], Mario Lusini[1], Francesco Santini[2] and Massimo Chello[1]

1 Unit of Cardiac Surgery, Università Campus Bio-Medico di Roma and Fondazione Policlinico Universitario Campus Bio-Medico, Rome, Italy

2 Unit of Cardiac Surgery, Università degli Studi di Genova and Ospedale Policlinico San Martino IRCCS, Genoa, Italy

*Address all correspondence to: a.nenna@policlinicocampus.it

References

[1] Jiang Y, Xu L, Liu Y, Deng B, Dong N, Chen S. Beating-heart on-pump coronary artery bypass grafting vs. off-pump coronary artery bypass grafting: A systematic review and meta-analysis. Journal of Thoracic Disease. 2021;**13**(7):4185-4194

[2] Wang W, Wang Y, Piao H, Li B, Wang T, Li D, et al. Early and medium outcomes of on-pump beating-heart versus off-pump CABG in patients with moderate left ventricular dysfunction. Brazilian Journal of Cardiovascular Surgery. 2019;**34**:62-69

[3] Phothikun A, Nawarawong W, Tantraworasin A, Phinyo P, Tepsuwan T. The outcomes of three different techniques of coronary artery bypass grafting: On-pump arrested heart, on-pump beating heart, and off-pump. PLoS One. 2023;**18**(5):e0286510

[4] Chan MJ, Lee CC, Chen SW, Tsai FC, Lin PJ, Fan PC, et al. Effect of different surgical type of coronary artery bypass grafting on kidney injury: A propensity score analysis. Medicine (Baltimore). 2017;**96**(45):e8395

[5] Zhu MZL, Huq MM, Billah BM, Tran L, Reid CM, Varatharajah K, et al. On-pump beating heart versus conventional coronary artery bypass grafting early after myocardial infarction: A propensity-score matched analysis from the ANZSCTS database. Heart, Lung & Circulation. 2019;**28**:1267-1276

[6] Wang C, Jiang Y, Jiang X, Chen S. On-pump beating heart versus conventional on-pump coronary artery bypass grafting on clinical outcomes: A meta-analysis. Journal of Thoracic Disease. 2021;**13**(7):4169-4184

[7] Dominici C, Salsano A, Nenna A, Spadaccio C, Mariscalco G, Santini F, et al. On-pump beating-heart coronary artery bypass grafting in high-risk patients: A systematic review and meta-analysis. Journal of Cardiac Surgery. 2020;**35**(8):1958-1978

[8] Tsai YT, Lin FY, Lai CH, Lin YC, Lin CY, Tsai CS. On-pump beating-heart coronary artery bypass provides efficacious short- and long-term outcomes in hemodialysis patients. Nephrology, Dialysis, Transplantation. 2012;**27**:2059-2065

[9] Munos E, Calderon J, Pillois X, Lafitte S, Ouattara A, Labrousse L, et al. Beating-heart coronary artery bypass surgery with the help of mini extracorporeal circulation for very high-risk patients. Perfusion. 2011;**26**:123-131

[10] Miyahara K, Matsuura A, Takemura H, Saito S, Sawaki S, Yoshioka T, et al. On-pump beating-heart coronary artery bypass grafting after acute myocardial infarction has lower mortality and morbidity. The Journal of Thoracic and Cardiovascular Surgery. 2008;**135**:521-526

[11] Ferrari E, Stalder N, von Segesser LK. On-pump beating heart coronary surgery for high risk patients requiring emergency multiple coronary artery bypass grafting. Journal of Cardiothoracic Surgery. 2008;**3**:38

[12] Rastan AJ, Eckenstein JI, Hentschel B, Funkat AK, Gummert JF, Doll N, et al. Emergency coronary artery bypass graft surgery for acute coronary syndrome: Beating heart versus conventional cardioplegic cardiac arrest strategies. Circulation. 2006;**114**:I477-I485

[13] Izumi Y, Magishi K, Ishikawa N, Kimura F. On-pump beating-heart coronary artery bypass grafting for acute myocardial infarction. The Annals of Thoracic Surgery. 2006;**81**:573-576

[14] Moscarelli M, Harling L, Attaran S, Ashrafian H, Casula RP, Athanasiou T. Surgical revascularisation of the acute coronary artery syndrome. Expert Review of Cardiovascular Therapy. 2014;**12**:393-402

[15] Prifti E, Bonacchi M, Giunti G, Frati G, Proietti P, Leacche M, et al. Does on-pump/beating-heart coronary artery bypass grafting offer better outcome in end-stage coronary artery disease patients? Journal of Cardiac Surgery. 2000;**15**:403-410

[16] Xia L, Ji Q, Song K, Shen J, Shi Y, Ma R, et al. Early clinical outcomes of on-pump beating-heart versus off-pump technique for surgical revascularization in patients with severe left ventricular dysfunction: The experience of a single center. Journal of Cardiothoracic Surgery. 2017;**12**:11

[17] Erkut B, Dag O, Kaygin MA, Senocak M, Limandal HK, Arslan U, et al. On-pump beating-heart versus conventional coronary artery bypass grafting for revascularization in patients with severe left ventricular dysfunction: Early outcomes. Canadian Journal of Surgery. 2013;**56**:398-404

[18] Darwazah AK, Bader V, Isleem I, Helwa K. Myocardial revascularization using on-pump beating heart among patients with left ventricular dysfunction. Journal of Cardiothoracic Surgery. 2010;**5**:109

[19] Pegg TJ, Selvanayagam JB, Francis JM, Karamitsos TD, Maunsell Z, Yu LM, et al. A randomized trial of on-pump beating heart and conventional cardioplegic arrest in coronary artery bypass surgery patients with impaired left ventricular function using cardiac magnetic resonance imaging and biochemical markers. Circulation. 2008;**118**:2130-2138

[20] Kim HJ, Oh YN, Ju MH, Kim JB, Jung SH, Chung CH, et al. On-pump beating heart versus conventional coronary artery bypass grafting: Comparative study on early and long-term clinical outcomes. Journal of Thoracic Disease. 2018;**10**:2656-2665

[21] Antunes PE, Ferrao de Oliveira J, Prieto D, Coutinho GF, Correia P, Branco CF, et al. Coronary artery bypass surgery without cardioplegia: Hospital results in 8515 patients. European Journal of Cardio-Thoracic Surgery. 2016;**49**:918-925

[22] Narayan P, Rogers CA, Bayliss KM, Rahaman NC, Panayiotou N, Angelini GD, et al. On-pump coronary surgery with and without cardioplegic arrest: Comparison of inflammation, myocardial, cerebral and renal injury and early and late health outcome in a single-centre randomised controlled trial. European Journal of Cardio-Thoracic Surgery. 2011;**39**:675-683

[23] Mizutani S, Matsuura A, Miyahara K, Eda T, Kawamura A, Yoshioka T, et al. On-pump beating-heart coronary artery bypass: A propensity matched analysis. The Annals of Thoracic Surgery. 2007;**83**:1368-1373

[24] Hwang B, Williams ML, Tian DH, Yan TD, Misfeld M. Coronary artery bypass surgery for acute coronary syndrome: A network meta-analysis of on-pump cardioplegic arrest, off-pump, and on-pump beating heart strategies. Journal of Cardiac Surgery. 2022;**37**(12):5290-5299

[25] Ueki C, Sakaguchi G, Akimoto T, Ohashi Y, Sato H. On-pump beating-heart technique is associated with lower morbidity and mortality following coronary artery bypass grafting: A meta-analysis. European Journal of Cardio-Thoracic Surgery. 2016;**50**:813-821

[26] Chaudhry UA, Harling L, Sepehripour AH, Stavridis G, Kokotsakis J, Ashrafian H, et al. Beating-heart versus conventional on-pump coronary artery bypass grafting: A meta-analysis of clinical outcomes. The Annals of Thoracic Surgery. 2015;**100**:2251-2260

Chapter 8

Secondary Prevention of Coronary Artery Disease

Joseph A. Moutiris

Abstract

Cardiovascular atherosclerotic disease (CvAD) and its consequences, coronary artery disease (CAD) and cerebrovascular disease (CvD), remain the major cause of morbidity and mortality in all countries. Addressing the predisposing factors related to lifestyle, such as smoking, lipid-rich diet, excessive stress, and lack of exercise, is important for primary and secondary prevention. In addition, the systematic use of cardioprotective medications, such as antiplatelets, statins, beta-blockers, and angiotensin-converting enzyme inhibitors, as well as new generation antidiabetics, for appropriate control, based on recent guidelines, of blood pressure, plasma glucose and lipid levels, lead to a further decrease in the risk for secondary cardiovascular events including cardiovascular death.

Keywords: coronary artery disease, secondary prevention, lipids, hypertension, diabetes, smoking, obesity

1. Introduction

The incidence and mortality of cardiovascular atherosclerotic disease (CvAD) and its clinical consequences, coronary artery disease (CAD) and cerebrovascular disease (CvD), although declining in some countries, due to better understanding of the predisposing risks and to the introduction of newer and more effective cardioprotective therapies, they are still considered a major cause of morbidity and mortality, influencing negatively the health systems of most countries [1].

Primary and secondary prevention of cardiovascular atherosclerotic disease, through adaptation of a healthy lifestyle, is an important part of the overall management. This includes avoidance of smoking, by preventing initiation or by cessation, of salt and of saturated lipids. In addition, engagement in regular physical activity and exercise programs, either in organized group rehabilitation settings, or as a lone approach, maintenance of a normal body weight, blood pressure, plasma glucose, and lipid levels, are important primary and secondary prevention measures [2].

Prevention of cardiovascular events in persons with established coronary artery disease is the topic of this chapter.

IntechOpen

2. The risk factors

The main cardiovascular risk factors are: cigarette smoking, hypertension, diabetes, obesity, and elevated total and LDL cholesterol.

2.1 Smoking

Chronic smokers carry a higher risk for cardiovascular disease, lung disease, and cancer than nonsmokers [3]. Moreover, it has been observed in large-scale surveys that approximately 18-30% of patients continue smoking after their first cardiovascular event. The percentage of active smokers at the time of consultation, in EUROASPIRE III, was 18.2%, nearly one in every five patients [4]. In EUROASPIRE IV, the prevalence of persistent smoking among patients who were smoking prior to the coronary event was 49.3%, despite the fact that most patients reported an intention to quit smoking [5]. Smoking cessation recommendations are shown in **Table 1**.

Quitting smoking after a cardiovascular event is important to reduce new events and mortality [6]. It is perhaps the most effective prevention measure reducing both the occurrence of myocardial infarction and death [7]. A chronic smoker who quits may gain some weight, up to 5 kg. However, the benefits overweigh the small risk of gaining weight [8]. Patients restarting smoking are usually those who suffer from some degree of depression related to their cardiovascular event. The approach of these patients must be different since they may need psychological support in addition to medical counseling and therapies [9].

2.2 Lipids

It is known that key role in atherogenesis plays the entry of oxidized LDL into the arterial wall [10]. Clinical trials have evidenced that reduction of LDL levels, with lipid-lowering drugs, reduces the risk of cardiovascular atherosclerotic disease [11]. There is no lower limit for LDL, presently, and no J-curve phenomenon has been observed so far, therefore the principle "the lower the better," seems to apply to explain the relation between LDL levels and the risk for cardiovascular atherosclerotic disease.

LDL can be measured directly, or it can be calculated using the Friedewald formula [12]. The calculation is valid when triglycerides are less than 400 mg (4.5 mmol/L). If more, then direct measurement is advised.

In mmol/L: LDL = total cholesterol – HDL – (0.45 × triglycerides).

In mg/dL: LDL = total cholesterol – HDL – (0.2 × triglycerides).

The Martin-Hopkins equation can be used instead to improve Friedewald estimation, especially in lower LDL groups [13].

The non-HDL level is another useful index to explain the cardiovascular risk [14]. It is calculated by subtracting HDL from total cholesterol, and it is not influenced by the LDL levels and can also be measured in the non-fasting state.

Recommendation	Class	Level
All smoking of tobacco should be stopped.	I	A
Smoking cessation is recommended regardless of weight gain.	I	A

Table 1.
Recommendations on smoking (ESC guidelines 2021).

Treating LDL is not an easy task. There are many drugs available with varying degree of tolerability and with some variations in the therapeutic effects [15]. The decision for initiation of therapy should be taken together with the patient since this will be life-long. Possible side effects should be explained carefully weighing the benefits for reducing the risk for events to the possible side effects.

Patients with established cardiovascular atherosclerotic disease should have their LDL levels below 55 mg/dL (1.4 mmol/L), whereas patients at high risk with multiple risks but without established cardiovascular disease should have their LDL lower than 70 mg/dL (1.8 mmol/L). Benefit has also been shown in patients who had their LDL lowered to less than 40 mg/dL (1.0 mmol/L). This is irrespective of gender or history of diabetes [16].

Regarding triglycerides, it is advised that their concentration should not exceed 150 mg/dL (1.7 mmol/L) as higher values may indicate an increased risk for events [17].

Achieving high levels of HDL is desired, and it is advised that this is done mainly with lifestyle measures, such as physical activity, rather than with drugs.

Secondary causes for dyslipidemias should always be addressed and if present, treated, although in patients with established CvAD administration of lipid-lowering drugs is recommended despite presence or not of secondary causes. Conditions, which may influence the lipid metabolism, include thyroid disease, hepatic disorders, renal disease, and Cushing syndrome [18].

It is known from epidemiological studies that high consumption of fish, vegetables, fruits, nuts, and whole grains, and lower consumption of red meat, processed food, saturated fat, carbohydrates, and salt are related to lower cardiovascular events [19].

Lipid-lowering medications include 3-hydroxy-3-methylglutaryl-coenzyme A reductase inhibitors, bile acid sequestrants, cholesterol gastrointestinal absorption inhibitors (ezetimibe), and PCSK9 inhibitors [20].

Statins are effective lipid-lowering drugs in reducing the levels of LDL, reducing hence the risk for a new event including cardiovascular mortality. They may also reduce triglycerides and increase HDL. Statins are considered first-line treatment in patients with chronic CvAD. Among the most frequent side effects of statin administration is myopathy in varying degree. Rhabdomyolysis is a rare side effect and needs immediate interruption of statin. Temporary rise in the hepatic enzymes has been observed in some patients. This is reversible in most cases. A few patients complain of weight gain. In general, statins are quite safe drugs with significant cardioprotective effects [21].

In patients not achieving the goals, ezetimibe, a cholesterol-absorption inhibitor, may be added. This causes further reduction in LDL [22]. Ezetimibe is considered as a second-line lipid-lowering drug, either in combination with a statin or alone if statins are not tolerated [22].

A newer group of lipid-lowering drugs are proprotein convertase subtilisin/kexin type 9 inhibitors (PCSK9 inhibitors). These monoclonal antibodies are considered very effective in reducing LDL. They are prescribed in addition to the maximum tolerated dose of statins plus ezetimibe, or when statins are not tolerated. There are currently two PCSK9 inhibitors approved by the FDA: Repatha (Evolocumab) and Praluent (Alirocumab). Administered subcutaneously every 2–4 weeks, the PCSK9 antibodies evolocumab and alirocumab reduce LDL by up to 60% in a broad range of populations. Two large cardiovascular outcome trials involving a total of 46,000 cardiovascular high-risk patients on guideline-recommended lipid-lowering therapy showed that treatment with evolocumab and alirocumab led to a relative reduction of cardiovascular risk by 15% after 2.2 and 2.8 years of treatment, respectively [23]. It seems that they also have an effect of triglycerides, on Lp(a), and on HDL.

Recommendation	Class	Level
It is recommended that a high-intensity statin is prescribed up to the highest tolerated dose to reach the LDL goals set for the specific risk group.	I	A
In patients with established cardiovascular atherosclerotic disease lipid-lowering treatment with an ultimate LDL goal of <55 mg/dL (1.4 mmol/L) and a > 50% reduction in LDL vs. baseline is recommended.	I	A
For secondary prevention patients not achieving their goals on a maximum tolerated dose of a statin plus ezetimibe, combination therapy including a PCSK9 inhibitor is recommended.	I	A

Table 2.
Recommendations in lipid therapy (ESC guidelines 2021).

Inclisiran is a long-acting hepatic PCSK9 synthesis inhibitor, known as siRNA (small interfering RNA interference). It works differently from the PCSK9 inhibitors by interrupting the "printing" of PCSK9 protein from the messenger RNA. It is also given twice yearly, whereas the others are given every two weeks. Inclisiran, given twice yearly, is associated with a reduction in LDL levels by 47.5% and 44.2%, after 210 days and 4 years, respectively [24]. The recommendations for lipid-lowering therapy are shown in **Table 2**.

2.3 Hypertension

A number of studies have correlated hypertension with a new event and with increased mortality in patients with CvAD [25–27]. Hypertension is defined as elevated blood pressure, systolic, diastolic, or both [28]. Although the upper acceptable limits of systolic and diastolic blood pressure are 140 and 90 mmHg, respectively, these may differ in relation to the way the measurement is done. For example, in the ambulatory BP measurement, the upper mean limits of normal are 130 and 80 mmHg, and home measurements are up to 135 and 85 mmHg, respectively [29]. These are shown in **Table 3**. **Table 4** shows the recommended values of BP in different clinical conditions in patients with diabetes, chronic kidney disease, coronary disease, and stroke.

2.4 Diabetes

In the EUROASPIRE IV survey [30], conducted in 24 European countries, among patients with coronary artery disease and less than 80 years old, 26.8% of the participants reported having diabetes and 37.6% had a BMI above 30. This high prevalence of diabetes and obesity indicates the need for intensive secondary approach including both lifestyle and adherence to cardioprotective medications, including the newer SGLT2i, in an attempt to reduce morbidity and mortality. **Table 5** summarizes the recommendation for the treatment of patients with diabetes.

3. Cardiac rehabilitation

Every patient having an acute cardiovascular event should undergo short- and long-term cardiac rehabilitation. This is an intervention, which needs the participation of many professionals, including cardiologists, nurses, exercise physiologists,

Category	SBP (mmHg)		DBP (mmHg)
Office BP	≥140	and/or	≥90
Ambulatory BP			
Daytime (or awake) mean	≥135	and/or	≥85
Night-time (or asleep) mean	≥120	and/or	≥70
24-h mean	≥130	and/or	≥80

Table 3.
Definitions of hypertension (ESC guidelines 2021).

Age group	Office SBP treatment target ranges (mmHg)				
	Hypertension	+ DM	+ CKD	+ CAD	+ Stroke/TIA
18 – 69 years	120–130	120–130	<140–130	120–130	120–130
	Lower SBP acceptable if tolerated				
≥70 years	<140 mmHg, down to 130 mmHg if tolerated				
DBP treatment	<80 for all treated patients				

Table 4.
Blood pressure target values in various clinical conditions (ESC guidelines 2021).

Recommendation	Class	Level
It is recommended that in persons with type 2 diabetes and cardiovascular atherosclerotic disease, the use of GLP-1RA or $SGLT_2$ inhibitor with proven outcome benefits is recommended to reduce cardiovascular and/or cardiorenal outcomes.	I	A

Table 5.
Recommendations for the treatment of patients with diabetes (ESC guidelines 2021).

Recommendation	Class	Level
Participation in a medically supervised, structured, cardiac rehabilitation program for patients after an atherosclerotic cardiovascular event and/or revascularization, and for patients with heart failure (mainly HFrEF) is recommended to improve patient outcomes.	I	A

Table 6.
Recommendations for cardiac rehabilitation (ESC guidelines 2021).

psychologists, and dieticians. Participation in rehabilitation programs is associated with an improvement in the quality of life, a reduction in hospitalizations, and in mortality [31].

Cardiac rehabilitation is not applied uniformly across Europe. In some countries, participation reaches the high 90%, whereas in other countries participation is negligible or absent.

Some general rules should apply for an effective rehabilitation program. Firstly, it must start the day after the acute cardiovascular event, for example, an acute myocardial infarction. It must be supervised by cardiologist and carried out by trained health professionals. The sessions and the time for each session should be individualized, but some general rules regarding a minimum time should be taken into consideration. All recognized cardiovascular risks should be addressed during rehabilitation. The European Association of Preventive Cardiology has set minimal and optimal standards for effective secondary prevention through cardiac rehabilitation [32]. The recommendations for cardiac rehabilitation are shown in **Table 6**.

4. The EUROASPIRE surveys

Since cardiovascular atherosclerotic disease (CvAD) remains the leading cause of disability and death across the globe, the main objectives of prevention is to reduce morbidity and mortality. Observational studies and randomized controlled trials, with lifestyle modification and pharmaceutical interventions, have evidenced a favorable influence of the known cardiovascular risk factors, on morbidity and mortality, and on preservation of the quality of life, in patients at high risk or with established CvAD.

The Joint European Societies (JES) guidelines on cardiovascular disease prevention published from 1994 to 2016 defined the lifestyle and risk factor goals for patients with coronary disease: give up smoking, choose healthy food, be physically active, have a body mass index (BMI) of less than 25 kg/m^2, and blood pressure of <140/90 mmHg (<130/80 mmHg if diabetes is present, a LDL cholesterol of <70 mg/dL (<1.8 mmol/L) or at least 50% reduction from baseline, glycated hemoglobin (HbA1c) <7.0% in the presence of diabetes, and appropriate use of cardioprotective medications which include: aspirin and other antiplatelets, β-blockers, angiotensin-converting enzyme inhibitors (ACEi)/angiotensin II receptor blockers (ARBs), and statins.

The EUROASPIRE (European Action on Secondary and Primary Prevention by Intervention to Reduce Events) surveys are audits designed to assess the clinical outcome and the degree to which the guidelines on cardiovascular disease prevention are met in the European populations. The surveys started in 1995-1996 and until 2014, four surveys have been completed among nine countries (1995-6), fifteen countries (1999-0), twenty-two countries (2006-8), and twenty-six countries (2012-2014). The surveys described the lifestyle and the risk factor management in patients with established coronary artery disease.

The results of EUROASPIRE surveys I to IV demonstrated a high prevalence of modifiable risk factors and inappropriate use of pharmacotherapy for blood pressure and lipid control in patients with established cardiovascular disease.

Moreover, the EUROASPIRE V survey, conducted between 2016 and 2018, among patients from 29 countries, incorporated in addition an assessment of dysglycaemia (impaired fasting glycemia IFG, impaired glucose tolerance IGT, and new diabetes) and kidney function in all patients [33]. A total of 8261 patients (females 26%) were interviewed. Nineteen percent smoked and 55% of them were persistent smokers, 38% were obese (body mass index ≥30 kg/m^2), 59% were centrally obese (waist circumference: men ≥102 cm; women ≥88 cm), while 34% were physically inactive (physical activity less than 30 min less than 5 times a week). Forty-two percent had a blood pressure ≥ 140/90 mmHg (≥130/85 if diabetic), 71% had low-density lipoprotein cholesterol (≥70 mg/dL (≥1.8 mmol/L), and 29% reported having diabetes. Antiplatelets were prescribed in 93% of patients, beta-blockers in 81%, angiotensin-converting enzyme inhibitors/angiotensin receptor blockers in 75%, and statins in 80% [33].

5. Summary

The main risk factors for cardiovascular atherosclerotic disease are high total and LDL cholesterol, elevated blood pressure, smoking, psychological stress, uncontrolled or poorly controlled diabetes, and obesity. Risk factors are treated based on the goals set by the guidelines.

Regular physical activity is important in secondary prevention.

In general, a reduction of sedentary time and more involvement in activities is recommended for all adults for primary and secondary prevention. Cardiac rehabilitation is encouraged for all patients with established CvAD.

A diet poor in saturated fats and rich in vegetables and fruits lowers the risk of cardiovascular disease.

Maintaining a normal weight may influence favorably other risks such as elevated blood pressure and elevated total and LDL cholesterol, reducing, thus, the CvAD risk.

Mental healthcare, especially management of depression, improves the quality of life and reduces the risk for CvAD.

Stopping smoking reduces the CvAD risk in all persons. Assistance drug therapy and follow-up support should be used to encourage patients to stop smoking if difficulties are observed.

The levels of LDL should be lowered by the use of statins, ezetimibe, and/or PCSK9 inhibitors in all patients with CvAD aiming to achieve the goal of values less than 55 mg/dL (<1.4 mmol/L), or if not achieved, by a reduction of more than 50% compared to baseline.

Lifestyle interventions and antihypertensive drugs, such as beta-blockers, ACE inhibitors, or ARBs, are recommended to lower BP levels based on recent guidelines aiming to achieve levels of 120/80 mmHg or lower.

Antiplatelet therapy with aspirin is indicated in all patients with CvAD.

In patients with CvAD and diabetes, treatment of diabetes with a target of 6.5–7.5% HbA1c is recommended.

Table 7 summarizes the use of cardioprotective medications in CvAD.

Aspirin 75–100 mg is recommended for patients with a previous myocardial infarction or revascularization.	I	A
In patients with chronic coronary syndromes clopidogrel 75 mg daily is recommended, in addition to aspirin, for 6 months following coronary stenting, irrespective of stent type, unless a shorter duration is indicated (1–3 months) due to risk or occurrence of life-threatening bleeding.	I	A
ACE inhibitors (or ARB) are recommended if a patient has other conditions (e.g., heart failure, hypertension, or diabetes)	I	A
Beta–blockers are recommended in patients with left ventricular dysfunction or systolic heart failure.	I	A
In patients with established atherosclerotic cardiovascular disease oral lipid-lowering treatment with an ultimate LDL goal of <55 mg/dL (1.4 mmol/L) and a > 50% reduction in LDL vs. baseline is recommended.	I	A

Table 7.
Recommendations for cardioprotective medical therapy in patients with CvAD (ESC guidelines 2021).

Conflict of interest

The author declares no conflict of interest.

Author details

Joseph A. Moutiris
Medical School, University of Nicosia, Cyprus

*Address all correspondence to: moutiris.j@unic.ac.cy

References

[1] Vaduganathan M, Mensah G, Turco J, et al. The global burden of cardiovascular diseases and risk. Journal of the American College of Cardiology. 2022;**80**(25):2361-2371

[2] Delgado-Lista J, Alcala-Diaz J, Torres-Pena J, et al. Long-term secondary prevention of cardiovascular disease with a Mediterranean diet and a low-fat diet (CORDIOPREV): A randomized controlled trial. The Lancet. 2022;**399**(1038):1876-1885

[3] Samet JM. Tobacco smoking: The leading cause of preventable disease worldwide. Thoracic Surgery Clinics. 2013;**23**(2):103-112

[4] Kotseva K et al. EUROASPIRE III: A survey on the lifestyle, risk factors and use of cardioprotective drug therapies in coronary patients from 22 European countries. European Journal of Cardiovascular Prevention and Rehabilitation. 2009;**16**(2):121-137

[5] Kotseva K, Wood D, De Bacquer D, et al. EUROASPIRE IV: A European Society of Cardiology survey on the lifestyle, risk factor and therapeutic management of coronary patients from 24 countries. European Journal of Preventive Cardiology. Apr 2016;**23**(6):636-648

[6] U.S. Department of Health and Human Services. Smoking Cessation. A Report of the Surgeon General. Atlanta, GA: U.S. Department of Health and Human Services, Centers for Disease Control and Prevention, National Center for Chronic Disease Prevention and Health Promotion, Office on Smoking and Health; 2020. Available from: www.cdc.gov/tobacco

[7] Critchley JA, Capewell S. Mortality risk reduction associated with smoking cessation in patients with coronary heart disease: A systematic review. The Journal of the American Medical Association. 2003;**290**:86-97

[8] Hu Y, Zong G, Liu G, Wang M, et al. Smoking cessation, weight change, typer 2 diabetes and mortality. The New England Journal of Medicine. 2018;**379**:623-632

[9] Hartmann-Boyce J, Stead LF, Cahill K, Lancaster T. Efficacy of interventions to combat tobacco addiction: Cohrane update of 2013 reviews. Addiction. 2014;**109**:1414-1425

[10] Nielsen LB. Transfer of low density lipoprotein into the arterial wall and risk of atherosclerosis. Atherosclerosis. 1996;**123**(1-2):1-15

[11] Soran H, Dent R, Durrington P. Evidence-based goals in LDL-C reduction. Clinical Research in Cardiology. 2017;**106**(4):237-248

[12] Krishnaveni P, Gowda VM. Assessing the validity of friedewald's formula and anandraja's formula for serum LDL-cholesterol calculation. Journal of Clinical and Diagnostic Research. 2015;**9**(12):BC01-BC04

[13] Martin SS, Blaha MJ, Elshazly MB, et al. Comparison of a novel method vs the Friedewald equation for estimating low-density lipoprotein cholesterol levels from the standard lipid profile. The Journal of the American Medical Association. 2013;**310**:2061-2068

[14] Packard CJ, Saito Y. Non-HDL cholesterol as a measure of atherosclerotic risk. Journal of

Atherosclerosis and Thrombosis. 2004;**11**(1):6-14

[15] Dayar E, Pechanova O. Targeted strategy in lipid-lowering therapy. Biomedicines. 2022;**10**(5):1090

[16] Bandyopadhyay D, Qureshi A, Ghosh S, Ashish K, Heise LR, Hajra A, et al. Safety and efficacy of extremely low LDL-cholesterol levels and its prospects in Hyperlipidemia management. Journal of Lipid Research. 2018;**23**(2018):859805

[17] Singh AK, Singh R. Triglyceride and cardiovascular risk: A critical appraisal. Indian Journal of Endocrinology and Metabolism. 2016;**20**(4):418-428

[18] Mosca S, Araújo G, Costa V, Correia J, Bandeira A, Martins E, et al. Dyslipidemia diagnosis and treatment: Risk stratification in children and adolescents. Journal of Nutrition and Metabolism. 21 Feb 2022;**2022**:4782344. DOI: 10.1155/2022/4782344

[19] Mozaffarian D. Natural trans fat, dairy fat, partially hydrogenated oils and cardiometabolic health: The Ludwigshafen risk and cardiovascular health study. European Heart Journal. 2016;**37**:1079-1081

[20] Chhetry M, Jialal I. Lipid-lowering drug therapy. In: StatPearls. Treasure Island (FL): StatPearls Publishing; 2023. Available from: https://www.ncbi.nlm.nih.gov/books/NBK541128

[21] Ruscica M, Ferri N, Banach M, Sirtori CR, Corsini A. Side effects of statins: From pathophysiology and epidemiology to diagnostic and therapeutic implications. Cardiovascular Research. 2023;**118**(17):3288-3304

[22] Shaya FT, Sing K, Milam R, Husain F, Del Aguila MA, Patel MY. Lipid-lowering efficacy of ezetimibe in patients with atherosclerotic cardiovascular disease: A systematic review and meta-analyses. American Journal of Cardiovascular Drugs. 2020;**20**(3):239-248

[23] Katzmann JL, Gouni-Berthold I, Laufs U. PCSK9 inhibition: Insights from clinical trials and future prospects. Frontiers in Physiology. 2020;**11**:595819, 2020

[24] Ray KK, Troquay RPT, Visseren FLJ, Leiter LA, Scott Wright R, Vikarunnessa S, et al. Long-term efficacy and safety of inclisiran in patients with high cardiovascular risk and elevated LDL cholesterol (ORION-3): Results from the 4-year open-label extension of the ORION-1 trial. The Lancet Diabetes & Endocrinology. 2023;**11**(2):109-119

[25] Yan J, Zhou J, Huang J, Zhang H, Deng Z, Du Y. The outcomes of acute myocardial infarction patients comorbidity with hypertension and hyperhomocysteinemia. Scientific Reports. 2021;**11**(1):22936

[26] Rakugi H, Yu H, Kamitani A, Nakamura Y, Ohishi M, Kamide K, et al. Links between hypertension and myocardial infarction. American Heart Journal. 1996;**13**:213-221

[27] Kobalava Z, Kvasnikov B, Burtsev Y. PRIDE study investigators. Effectiveness and tolerability of bisoprolol/perindopril single-pill combination in patients with arterial hypertension and a history of myocardial infarction: The PRIDE observational study. Advances in Therapy. 2023;**40**(6):2725-2740

[28] Giles TD, Materson BJ, Cohn JN, Kostis JB. Definition and classification of hypertension: An update, The Journal of Clinical Hypertension. 2009;**11**(11):611-614

[29] Schutte AE, Kollias A, Stergiou GS. Blood pressure and its variability: Classic and novel measurement techniques. Nature Reviews. Cardiology. 2022;**19**(10):643-654

[30] Kotseva K, Wood D, De Bacquer D, De Backer G, Rydén L, Jennings C, et al. EUROASPIRE Investigators. EUROASPIRE IV: A European Society of Cardiology survey on the lifestyle, risk factor and therapeutic management of coronary patients from 24 European countries. European Journal of Preventive Cardiology. 2016;**23**(6):636-648

[31] Taylor RS, Dalal HM, McDonagh STJ. The role of cardiac rehabilitation in improving cardiovascular outcomes. Nature Reviews Cardiology. 2022;**19**(3):180-194

[32] Ambrosetti M, Abreu A, Corrà U, Davos CH, Hansen D, Frederix I, et al. Secondary prevention through comprehensive cardiovascular rehabilitation: From knowledge to implementation. 2020 update. A position paper from the Secondary Prevention and Rehabilitation Section of the European Association of Preventive Cardiology. European Journal of Preventive Cardiology. 2021;**28**(5):460-495

[33] Kotseva K, De Backer G, De Bacquer D, et al. Lifestyle and impact on cardiovascular risk factor control in coronary patients across 27 countries: Results from the European Society of Cardiology ESC-EORP EUROASPIRE V registry. European Journal of Preventive Cardiology. 2019;**26**(8):824-835. DOI: 10.1177/2047487318825350